THE
ACCESSORY
HANDBOOK

---

*A Costume Designer's Secrets for Buying,
Wearing, and Caring for Accessories*

ALISON FREER

Illustrations by Julia Kuo

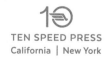

TEN SPEED PRESS
California | New York

CONTENTS

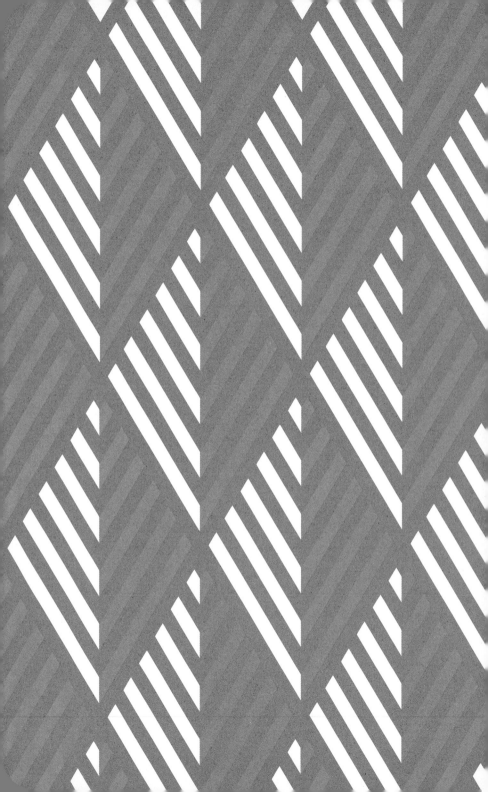

INTRODUCTION

WANT GREAT STYLE? ACCESSORIZE!

I once worked with the incredible Mr. T on a music video shoot. I was the costume designer for the project, but T didn't actually need my help at all—he had already accessorized himself for the occasion with a giant (solid gold, mind you) plate, fork, spoon, and knife around his neck on four separate golden chains. And when I say giant, I mean it was a full-sized dinner plate and silverware set—the plate alone was ten inches across. I asked him, "T, why are you wearing a life-sized gold dinner plate and silverware around your neck?" He immediately shot back with his answer (in his gravelly Mr. T voice): "Alison, I'm try-ing to tell Hollywood, 'LET'S DO LUNCH!'"

I understood exactly what Mr. T was getting at—because accessories are power. They're magic. They are a way to express your personal style—and to let everyone know what you happen to be thinking about or feeling on any particular day. Accessories take you from simply wearing clothes to actually being dressed. They are armor with which to fight the world—a sort of talisman against anything that could possibly hurt you. For example: when I'm feeling like I need a shot of confidence, I grab my most blingy necklace (one that spells B-A-D in rhinestones)—and suddenly I pity the fool who would dare mess with me.

It's tempting to write off the idea of accessories as frivolous and needless, but every accessory first existed as the answer to a real human need. Since the dawn of time, if you had to carry something bigger than your own two hands, you needed a bag. A diamond ring was portable wealth that women could carry at all times; umbrellas are mobile shelters; pins and brooches held capes and jackets closed long before buttons became *a thing*; and belts handily carried swords for easy access. Most people don't feel the need to keep a sword close at hand these days (though if you choose to, I won't judge), but the right accessory can still be a lifesaver: a good cross body bag leaves your arms free to fend off possible attackers, a light scarf will keep you toasty warm in an overly air-conditioned office; and a fierce cocktail ring provides a conversational jumping-off point in an awkward social situation.

Accessories, as the name itself implies, are accessible to everyone. It doesn't matter what age, shape, or size you are (or even the size of your wallet), there's an accessory out there that will complement, fit, and totally elevate your existing look. Accessories are the great equalizer—true democracy in fashion. Inexpensive clothes can sometimes look poorly made, but a cheap bauble can look like a million bucks when worn in an interesting way. That little scrap of ribbon you're wearing around your neck could be Chanel, for all anyone knows. Accessories are usually a far better investment than clothing, because you can spend a measly five dollars, wind up looking great, and nobody will ever be the wiser. Plus, they take up way less space than clothes do—so they're far easier to store. Accessories even transcend eras—and a bauble from eighty years ago can look fresh and new when paired with a modern garment.

Accessories are also the number one way you can easily change up your look. A tailored business suit worn with elegant gold jewelry and law office–appropriate shoes can take on a glam-rock, David Bowie–inspired edge when paired with metallic ankle boots and a pile of candy-colored gemstone necklaces. A dress you've worn almost a thousand times can seem like an entirely different one when you belt it and add an armful of jangling bracelets. Trading your neutral bag for an unusual colored or patterned one is a great way to perk up your style in the dead of winter when you're stuck wearing the same bulky coat for months on end. And if you find yourself suddenly needing to wear your work clothes out to a bar, just swap your boring daytime heels for a pair of cool sneakers, switch out your day bag for one you'd never be able to fit your computer in, and scoop your hair up into a ball cap or beanie. You'll instantly look as if you planned it. Wearing accessories is all about creating visual interest, but figuring out how to make everything work in a harmonious way (without it feeling as if you suddenly decided to wear a novelty foam cowboy hat with your regular work outfit) can be a challenge.

Incorporating accessories into your everyday look (no matter where you're headed) is actually far easier than the fashion magazines make it out to be—because half the art of wearing accessories is just remembering to put them on in the first place. After all these years, I've finally trained myself to always take a minute before I leave the house to consider if I own an accessory that would work with what I'm wearing—and I instantly look more put together for it. Put a sticky note on your mirror to remind yourself to do the same, and it will soon become second nature for you too.

ALL YOU NEED IS A LITTLE CONFIDENCE

You'd think actors and celebrities were just innately confident about wearing accessories with panache, but in the years I've spent styling them for TV shows, commercials, and music videos, they are always telling me how much they love accessories—yet they still feel as if they don't exactly know what to do with them. This reaction consistently stuns me, because on the face of it, it's rather simple: put the accessory of your choice on your body. Congrats! You are now wearing an accessory. What I think all those accessory-phobic celebs are really saying is that, yes, even they lack the confidence to successfully wear and style accessories. You may not realize it, but personal style is actually just 90 percent confidence—that other 10 percent comes from the accessories you wear.

Mr. T already knew one of the main keys to wearing accessories with confidence: always have an answer ready for why you are wearing a certain something in the first place. Thinking about it in advance ensures you have something to say to those rude piglets who try to drain your confidence by constantly questioning your accessory choices. It's hard to be brave and try something new when you know that a bunch of boring office drones are of course going to comment on it. So when someone scoffs, "Why do you always wear a scarf around your neck?", hit 'em with your preplanned answer: "Because it's the most effective sunscreen there is!" When cross-examined about your oversized floral beaded necklace, a simple "I just love flowers!" will do. If questioned about your eccentric shoe choices while you're killing it in a pair of leopard-print platform shoes, responding, "I'm a very dramatic individual, you know!" will suffice. If you get caught off-guard, you can fall back on the old standby: "Because it makes me happy!" And, as a bonus, forcing yourself to think about why you truly love certain accessories will make it way easier to pick out pieces that suit you in the first place.

Having a ready response to naysayers is a good idea, but the real secret to wearing accessories with confidence lies in simple experimentation. Trial and error is the key to getting into the accessory-wearing groove—and not being afraid to perhaps look a little silly almost always pays off in the end. Obviously, don't wear a giant gold dinner plate à la Mr. T to a job interview unless you know you can pull it off, but if it's just a trip to the mall or a fun night out with your best pals, you've got nothing to lose by trying an accessory trend that may be old news for some—but totally new for you.

If you're at all afraid of wearing something unfamiliar that you may deem a little crazy, remember this: what's the worst that can happen? Jan from accounting (or someone at the gas station) thinks you look silly? I'm pretty sure they'll live through it. And if you change your mind or become self-conscious about whatever accessory you're wearing, you can always just take off the offending item and shove it in your pocket or purse. But if you think you may wind up taking off a smallish accessory (such as earrings, a bracelet, or a ring) while out for the day, be sure to carry along an empty zipper lock sandwich bag to put it in. That way, you lessen the chance of losing it—as a piece of jewelry corralled in a sandwich bag calls more attention to itself than if it were just floating around by itself in your pocket or purse, and is therefore way less likely to be overlooked. The sandwich bag trick is every costume designer's secret for making sure actors who remove their personal jewelry on set don't just stick it in their pockets, forget about it, and then lose it to the laundry.

BUT REALLY, WHAT'S THE SECRET?

People are forever asking me what the secret formula is for wearing jewelry and accessories in ways that seem natural and unforced—as if I'm somehow the Albert Einstein of Accessories. They know that accessories are the key to looking truly stylish, but they can't quite crack the code for wearing them without feeling as if the accessories are drawing attention in a distracting, disjointed way. But what works—and what is way too much—is different for every individual. There are no big secrets or one-size-fits-all formulas for wearing accessories successfully, and anyone who tells you differently is lying.

It just takes a little time, energy, and desire to get it right—and I promise, you are already more put together than you are likely giving yourself credit for. Just because someone spent hours getting dressed doesn't mean they have great personal style. On the flip side, someone who is plain (or a little bit messy, even!) can still be stylish. There's no single or *right* way to wear and enjoy accessories, but absolutely everyone can benefit from them. It can be as simple as tossing on a crazily colorful pair of shoes with a basic outfit you've already worn a million times—or trading in your ho-hum everyday bag for one that truly expresses your personality.

Wearing accessories that you love can instantly lift you up and make you smile back at yourself in the mirror when you're feeling down. And if you're the type of person who saves your fancy accessories for a special occasion, why not make every day special? Why not make every day a celebration of yourself? Why not wear the things you feel your best in? In other words: just do it!

Style (and a knack for wearing accessories) isn't something you just have to be born with or tough luck to you, kid—it can be learned. Believe me, I didn't have the best sense of style when I started out as a costume designer! But once I set my mind to it, I became attuned to the things that inspired me: bright colors, zany prints, always a little shine and sparkle, and layers of fun accessory details. Now, the looks I put together for the TV shows I style all bear my signature—they are forever colorful, cheeky, joyful, and alive.

I'll attempt to give you some formulas here for what works for most accessory-wearing folks, but the truth is there are always exceptions. I can give you a road map—a blueprint, really—for how to wear accessories in a way that feels fun, fresh, and most importantly, enhances the beauty you've already got, but it will take you only so far. Once you start paying attention to what you like and what sparks your interest, you'll write your own road map—and it will all start to come together naturally. With time (and a little practice), you'll start to understand how to wear accessories in a way that brings you joy and truly enhances who you are. One day, not so long from now, you'll put on an accessory—and just know that it's right for you.

If you feel overwhelmed, take heart: nobody assembles a proper accessory wardrobe in a day, a week, a month, or even a year. It's a process—and it's ever-changing. You may be really into pearls and heels one week—then Birkenstocks and wooden beads the next. Some weeks, you may feel the urge to wear pearls and Birkenstocks together! You have to give yourself the time to think about, develop, and hone your aesthetic instincts. It definitely takes a bit of work, especially if you are used to just purchasing and wearing whatever you think is currently cool, hip, or "in." That's not to say that you should never try anything trendy—just that the trendy things you try should still be something that speaks to your style and unique personality.

If you're not used to wearing accessories at all, a good way to test the waters is to start adding a single accessory to whatever you're wearing, even if you're just staying home. If you already own a fair number of accessories but aren't sure how to start styling them, a great trick is to pick one accessory that you love (a pair of silver shoes, a giant gold skull ring, or your grandmother's watch) and build a look around it—letting the accessory be the focal point of your outfit. If your accessory issue is that you've already worn every-thing you own and are bored of it all, what you may need is a little inspiration—so search out photos of people wearing similar accesso-ries to see how they chose to style them. Even after dressing people professionally for close to twenty years—in addition to writing two books and countless articles on fashion—I'm still forever going online to look up stuff like "How to wear men's-style shoes + fashion blog-gers" or "Ways to wear a clutch with jeans + stylist secrets." It's not that I don't have my own ideas, but fresh, new, interesting ways to wear accessories are always popping up.

Once you start paying attention, an accessory style will eventually speak to you, inspire you, and start to unlock the real you. Practice and persistence—not some magical "she's born with it" gene—make perfect. When you begin to understand which accessories truly express your individuality, you'll be off to the races—never to leave the house un-accessorized ever again. And remember: everybody, including Mr. T, had to start their accessory journey somewhere.

HOW MUCH IS TOO MUCH?

Since I was old enough to walk, I have heard that dumb advice about taking one accessory off before you leave the house, lest you look as if you're wearing way too much stuff. Not only is this advice outdated, it's just plain wrong. The best thing about dabbling in accessories to change up your look is that you don't always have to be the same person every day. You can pare down your accoutrements on Monday to be a sleek minimalist—then pile on as many bangles as your arms will hold on a Tuesday and be the best version of Iris Apfel you possibly can. If it starts to feel like a total costume (meaning the accessories are wearing you instead of the other way around), it might actually be true that you have on a little too much stuff. But really, you are the best judge of this, not some boring old advice from fashion fogeys that we've all heard a million times.

THE MASTER SHOT

A good way to approach wearing accessories is to think like a costume designer—which means you'll want to carefully consider how each accessory works as part of your entire ensemble. If you watch many films, you'll start to notice that most scenes open with a "master shot" that establishes location and setting—and presents a character's look from head to toe for the first time. The master shot is important in real life too, because while a lot of old-fashioned sayings are just that— old-fashioned—it's still true that first impressions are everything.

One of the most style-centric master shots in history focuses exclusively on Audrey Hepburn's iconic look as Holly Golightly in the opening scene of *Breakfast at Tiffany's*. The camera lovingly follows her entire look as she hops out of the cab and walks towards the store, gazing in the windows as she eats a Danish and drinks coffee: the simple black shoes followed the mermaid swoop of her long black sheath dress (designed by Hubert de Givenchy), the elbow-length gloves, the quintuple-strand of pearls dangling down her back and gathered at the front with a large rhinestone flower, the dark tortoiseshell Oliver Goldsmith sunglasses, and the tiny bejeweled tiara that topped off her hairdo. Every one of those accessories was important on its own, but together they worked in concert to take a simple black dress from ho-hum to legendary. Holly's look in that master shot holds up amazingly well all those years later—and it's largely due to the careful choosing of accessories that flowed flawlessly from head to toe.

Every time you walk into a room—be it at a party, dinner date, or job interview—it's a chance to stage your own master shot, to consider how your entire ensemble and chosen accessories look when viewed from top to bottom: the way your shoes, belt, handbag, jewelry, and eyeglasses work in concert. This may sound hard to achieve, but it's really not. All you need to do is invest in a full-length mirror if you don't already have one, because the key to looking good from head-to-toe is actually being able to see your whole look. You can only see so much of your outfit when you're standing hunched over the toilet, trying to look in your tiny medicine cabinet mirror. Being able to view and consider (from all angles) how your accessories play with the clothing you've selected is the key to making a masterful grand entrance—and as always, practice makes perfect.

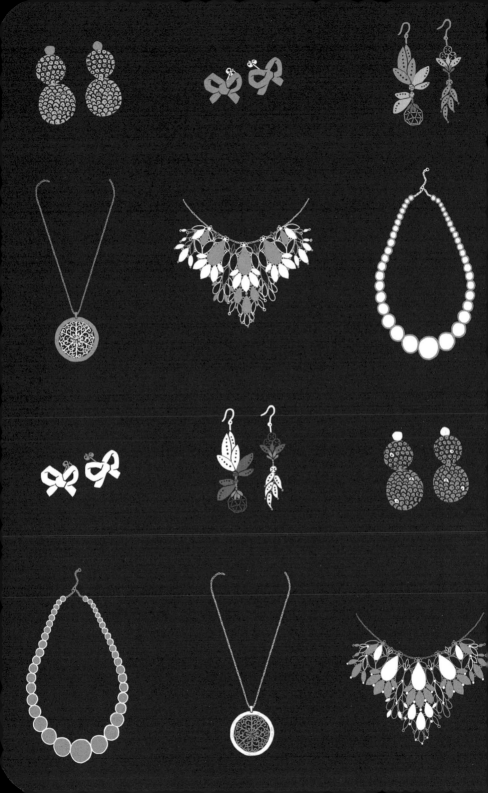

CHAPTER 1

JEWELRY

The Backbone of Accessorizing

The idea of jewelry is actually a bit silly when you think about it. Why did humans ever chose to adorn themselves with gems, chains, crystals, and beads; invest them with meaning; and then have to navigate the world with all this stuff hanging off their bodies? The obvious answer is that jewelry has long been used to signal things like wealth, clan affiliation, family, religion, and marital or social status, but the main reason to wear it these days is to look cute—and get compliments. It also works to allow the wearer to express personality and individuality, but the sheer amount of jewelry out there can be overwhelming to sift through, so it's best to start your journey in your very own closet.

EVALUATE WHAT YOU ALREADY OWN

Assembling a jewelry wardrobe that works for you begins with taking a good, hard look at what you already own. Before you buy one more piece of jewelry, figure out which pieces you already own and wear—and ask yourself what it is you like about those particular pieces. Are they large, shiny, sparkly, and dazzling? Or are the pieces you wear most often smaller in size? Are they made of wood or ceramic? Or do you gravitate toward sparkles like a magpie?

If certain pieces from your existing jewelry collection consistently draw compliments from others, chances are those pieces have something about them that really works for you, whether it's complementing your facial shape, expressing your personality, or just bringing joy and uniqueness to your overall look. Take the time to explore why you think those things are working for you and learn to trust your instincts. Once you train your eye a bit, you'll start to spot jewelry-shaped spaces in your outfits: a boatnecked blouse will call out for a dangling pendant necklace; a flared sleeve will look unfinished until you add a chunky cuff bracelet; and a turtleneck will seem like a boring, endless expanse of fabric unless you top it with a pair of hoop earrings or some long chains to break up the look.

WHAT'S YOUR JEWELRY STYLE?

A common mistake people make is buying jewelry without considering how it fits in with the rest of their collection. Having a basic idea of your general style to guide you through the minefield of available jewelry options is a good way to never wind up with something you won't actually wear. You don't have to pick one signature jewelry style and stick with it, but it's worth identifying your basic style to inform future purchases. Below are a few common jewelry styles to get you thinking, but in time, you'll start to find and hone your own, highly personal jewelry aesthetic—and then always have it at the ready to decide if a piece is right for you.

THE CLASSIC

Think of Jacqueline Bouvier Kennedy Onassis' timeless look as she entertained dignitaries at the White House and walked the streets of New York City—and you'll have nailed classic jewelry style. Look for:

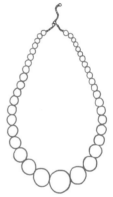

- » Elegant pearls

- » Understated diamond stud earrings

- » A simple leather-strapped watch

- » A bracelet with charms you've been collecting for years

THE ONE-OF-A-KIND

Legendary artist Frida Kahlo exemplified this style with her love for intricately handmade pieces from various regions of Mexico, a look she adopted after her 1929 marriage to Diego Rivera: a locket with river pearls from Oaxaca, a gold choker from Yucatán, and painstakingly wire-worked silver earrings from Sultepec and Toluca. Look for:

» Handmade necklaces strung with clay beads

» Woven string bracelets

» Wire-worked earrings

THE MAGPIE

If your signature jewelry style is the magpie, you'll know it. Think Rosalind Russell dripping with multiple statement pieces in *Auntie Mame*, and you're on the right track. Look for:

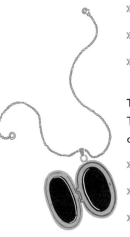

» Sparkling faux-gemstone bracelets

» Necklaces with quirky pendants as big as your head

» Fistfuls of rings that ooze character and charm

THE HEIRLOOM

The person who wears heirloom jewelry lives by the adage "Timeless—not trendy." Look for:

» Locket necklaces

» Monogrammed signet rings

» Pieces that have been handed down for generations

THE MODERN ART TEACHER

Ms. Frizzle from the classic animated show *The Magic School Bus* perfectly embodies the essence of this joyful, eclectic style. Look for:

» Geometric pieces

» Square bangle bracelets

» Abstractly shaped drop earrings

THE GLOBE-TROTTER

If anyone has ever taken a good look at your witchy, bohemian-tinged jewelry and made a Stevie Nicks reference, this is likely your signature jewelry style. Look for:

» Turquoise rings

» Crystal-studded bracelets

» Strands of multicolored agate beads

» Pieces with natural elements like wood or cork

THE MINIMALIST

Simple, minimalist jewelry doesn't have to mean boring—so if delicate pieces are your jam, embrace them. You can still be crazy stylish without having your jewelry scream at the top of its lungs. Look for:

» Delicate, weightless chain necklaces with a dainty pendant or charm

» Barely there silver or gold rings that add a tiny glint to the hands

» Thin hoop earrings or simple studs

NECKLACES: WHY AND HOW

Your head is the crown jewel of your body (and contains a lot of important information), so it makes sense that the piece of jewelry that best frames it, the necklace, is the single most popular piece of jewelry there is.

FOUR DIFFERENT WAYS TO WEAR THE SAME OLD NECKLACES

Wearing a necklace seems so simple: Place necklace on neck. Latch clasp. Congrats! You are now wearing a necklace. But nothing is ever really that easy, and chances are, you're a bit bored of the necklaces you already have in your closet. But don't toss them—try wearing them in one of these new, different ways instead:

STATEMENT: Surely you've heard a thousand fashion bloggers trumpet the outfit-changing genius of the statement necklace. Also called a bib necklace, this is a shorter necklace with front-dangling ornaments that somewhat resembles, well, a baby bib. It looks good with almost any garment—but for a fresh spin on what can easily become a tired look, try wearing one nestled underneath the collar of a button-front shirt or polo that is buttoned all the way up, giving it the effect of wearing a brooch at your throat.

CHOKER: Popularized by Princess Alexandra of England in the nineteenth century, chokers are tight-fitting necklaces (worn at the throat) that mimic a dog's collar. Chokers have come roaring back into fashion as of late—and show zero signs of ever going away again. Since they don't interfere with any garment's neckline (unless it's a turtleneck), chokers look good with pretty much everything. Chokers are also the ultimate DIY jewelry, because anything tied flatteringly around your neck counts as a choker—even a piece of leftover Christmas ribbon or a scrap of twine. You can also take a random charm that's been floating in your jewelry box forever and thread it onto a simple ribbon or string to give it a new lease on life. And if you think you are a person who can't wear a choker success-fully due to the size, width, or length of your neck, try again with the thinnest ribbon you can find—and wear it a little lower so that the charm settles into the hollow at the center of your neck, not farther up on your throat. I've yet to find a person this hasn't worked for.

PEARLS: A long rope of pearls that cascades down from the throat can easily veer into old-lady territory—but if you fold the strand in half and twist the ends around until it's short enough to wear at the throat, using a brooch or pin as a clasp to attach the two ends together at the front of your neck, you've instantly modernized it. If you're looking to turn a simple strand of short, smaller pearls into something with a dash of personality, lay the strand flat on a table and tie a simple knot roughly in the center of the strand before putting it on, giving an otherwise boring set of pearls a bit of an offbeat focal point—and making them the perfect foil for a rough-and-tumble flannel shirt, beat-up leather jacket, or old concert T-shirt with holes that needs a bit of ladylike style to perk it up.

CHAINS: Usually made of gold or silver-toned metal (think Mr. T), chains come in a variety of link styles (such as box, rope, Cuban, or snake) and widths (which are measured in millimeters). Chain necklaces look good with almost anything, but really make a statement when you pile a bunch of them on at once. (To get a jump on artfully wearing multiple chains at the same time, flip ahead to page 20.)

If a huge jumble of chains isn't your style, consider a thin, simple, metal chain that you can add charms to as time goes by. It's one of the most versatile jewelry pieces you can own. Just make sure to look for one with a slim-line clasp so you can slip charms on and off easily—or look for charms that come with their own spring clasps, meant to be quickly added and subtracted to whatever chain your heart desires.

WHY DOES MY CLASP KEEP SLIDING DOWN IN FRONT?

If you suffer from necklace clasps that constantly worm their way to the front where the pendant is, I'm sad to say there really isn't a foolproof solution to this problem. The reason it happens in the first place is that the clasp is too heavy for the chain and pendant combination, so its weight drags it down toward the lighter pendant in front. A ten dollar clasp extender that distributes the weight of the clasp more evenly, while anchoring it at the back of your neck, greatly helps, but it doesn't completely eradicate the problem.

DOES THIS REALLY NEED A NECKLACE?

Wearing a necklace is an ultra-easy way to add some spice to even the most boring outfit, but if your garment is already adorned with a fair amount of beading, ruffles, or other business happening, you likely don't need to add anything to it at all—since a necklace worn over something embellished is usually a bridge too far. The general rule is the gaudier the outfit, the more basic the necklace should be—while a simpler ensemble is license to go hog wild.

MATCH YOUR NECKLACE TO YOUR NECKLINE

Does your necklace always seem to interfere with your garment's neckline? The key to keeping things from looking too busy up top lies in balancing the distance between your neckline and the necklace. For example: if your neckline is lower (such as a strapless or scoop style), you'll likely want to keep your necklace above the top of the garment, ideally not touching it at all. Longer necklaces usually work better on higher-necked tops (such as turtlenecks or crew necks), since there is then no skin showing between the necklace and the neckline—so the overall look is cleaner and less cluttered to the eye. This may sound confusing, but here are a handful of common neckline shapes (and the likely best necklace style for each) to help you get the hang of things:

TURTLENECK: Despite what you may have heard, wearing a necklace over a turtleneck is A-OK. It just needs to be on the longer side (anywhere from twenty-four to thirty inches) to balance out the weight of so much fabric at the neck.

STRAPLESS: A necklace that sits right on your collarbone and has a bit of heft to it is the perfect foil to bare shoulders. Try a rounded, weighty, collar-style necklace that closely resembles something Cleopatra would have worn—it will draw every eye in the room to you immediately.

SQUARE: A top with a square neckline looks smoking with a square pendant that echoes its boxy shape, but any shape pendant will really do. If you want your necklace to be the star of your look, make sure the pendant doesn't dip any lower than your neckline.

SCOOP: A busy, elaborate necklace in a shorter U-shape will complement a scoop-necked garment perfectly, since this style of neckline won't get in the way of any dangling ornaments.

CREW NECK: A bib necklace works incredibly well when it's worn exactly as the name implies (as a bib)—so layer one on over a simple crew neck T-shirt or sweater for the full bib-like effect. It's a great way to add visual interest to what can tend to be a slightly boring neckline style.

BOATNECK: Long, graduated beads or chains look great when paired with a slightly off-the-shoulder boatneck top. The contrast between straight lines and curved edges is what gives this look lots of interest.

WEARING NECKLACES WHEN YOU HAVE BIG BOOBS

Wondering how to wear a necklace without having a giant arrow pointing to your ample cleavage? The key to making it work is paying close attention to where the necklace sits on your chest. You have to find your personal necklace sweet spot and then stick with it. Your sweet spot is likely higher than you think—as you'll want your necklace to hang above the point at which your boobs start to swell out. If any of the necklace-wearing scenarios below sounds familiar, wearing your necklaces a bit higher on your chest is probably the fix:

» Your necklace juts out over your bust and dangles in the air.

» Your necklace dangles down and comes to a rest in your cleavage.

» Your necklace sits on your bust as if it were sitting on a shelf.

Also, keep in mind that larger, chunkier necklaces worn closer to the throat usually work well for those with bounteous boob-age, since they draw the eye upward, making your neck and face the first thing people notice—not your chest.

NECKLACES FOR SHORTER NECKS

If you feel as if you have a short neck, try wearing longer necklaces—anywhere between twenty-four and thirty inches. They will lengthen your neck in an instant.

MORE, MORE, MORE: HOW TO STACK AND LAYER NECKLACES LIKE A CHAMP

The fastest way to feel like a fashion dolt is to attempt wearing multiple necklaces. It's way too easy to have it all go wrong, but it's also not quite as hard as it seems—it just takes time to get it right. As you practice, don't worry yourself too much about the inevitable slight overlapping of pieces. You can pretty much pile on any necklaces you like and be fine, but I'm going to give you a few cheat codes to lean on until you feel as if you know what you're doing.

KEEP IT ALL IN THE FAMILY: If you're new to wearing multiple necklaces, try sticking to pieces in the same color family. A cascade of all gold, all silver, or all black metal chains makes quick visual sense, making a stack of them look less busy than it really is. But keep in mind that mixing metals and textures is what really adds visual interest and makes a set of layered necklaces great. Think gold mixed with wood, plastic worn with natural agate, or pearls paired with rhinestones.

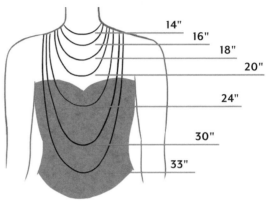

MIX LIGHT WITH HEAVY: An easy way to start your necklace layering journey is by placing your most delicate piece closest to your neck and cascading your heavier pieces down as you layer. Alternatively, you can start with one attention-grabbing centerpiece, plugging in two more bold necklaces on either side of it (meaning one that falls just above your main necklace—and one below it). Finish things off with a few light, simple chains of wood, beads, or stones, as they will add depth and interest to the whole look while making it clear that you did in fact mean to wear all those pieces together.

MAKE GOOD USE OF SPACE: The amount of empty space between each necklace doesn't have to match exactly, but make sure the necklaces don't lie directly on top of one another. Anywhere between one-half to one-inch spacing between necklaces is ideal. But if a little overlap is going to occur, it looks best when you confine it to your shortest pieces that are worn closest to your throat.

THE SAMPLE STACK: It's not mandatory, but using your heaviest, longest necklace as your bottom layer can help to anchor your entire look. This means that the perfect four-necklace stack would look something like this:

» First, a thin, delicate chain with a small pendant worn close to your throat—fourteen to sixteen inches is usually perfect.

» Next, go for a slightly longer metal chain (around eighteen inches), possibly with a medium-sized pendant that is under two inches in length.

» Below that, add in a beaded necklace (something in stone or wood would work well) around twenty-four inches in length.

» Finally, finish it off with a long, roughly thirty-inch chain with a pendant around two inches in length.

Obviously you can adjust, add, subtract, and improvise with your own layered necklace stacks—this is just a starting point. Once you really get going, there's almost no end to what you can successfully layer together. Just keep going until it finally looks right to your eye.

A QUICK FIX FOR PERFECT LAYERING

A good way to easily adjust necklace lengths in order to layer more effectively is to connect a simple chain bracelet to either end of your necklace's clasp in order to temporarily lengthen it. I've also used tiny gold safety pins to shorten or lengthen my chain-link necklaces for maximum layering options. Both options work like a charm, giving you lots of leeway to layer however you like.

HOW TO KEEP YOUR NECKLACES FROM GETTING TANGLED

If you have a tangled necklace that will just not come unknotted, try placing it on a clean plate (not one with last night's dinner on it) and sprinkling the knot with a bit of baby powder. It acts as a non-messy lubricant, and like magic, the knot will become a lot looser and can then be easily detangled with a needle or safety pin. Rinse or brush off any excess powder and you're good to go. If your chain necklaces tend to get mercilessly tangled while traveling (or while sitting in your drawer at home), start threading one side of your worst offenders through a disposable drinking straw. You can use multiple straws for longer necklaces or cut straws into smaller segments for shorter ones. If your necklace is on the thicker side, use a thicker straw, like a smoothie or bubble tea straw.

OUCH, MY HAIR!

If your hair tends to constantly get caught in your necklace clasp, try this slightly weird hack: buy a few inches of aquarium tube from a pet shop and snip off a tiny piece to cover the clasp. Slide it onto the chain and then scoot it over to cover the clasp mechanism after you've fastened it. This may seem like a lot of work, but having your hair ripped out by every single necklace you own is no picnic.

EARRINGS: WHY AND HOW

Earrings aren't just things to hang off your ears—the practice of piercing the earlobe for dangling ornaments actually dates back to at least the Bronze Age, when earrings were used to indicate the wearer's religious, political, or tribal identity. Earrings were also sometimes indicators of social status or as an unfortunate earmark for those who were enslaved. Earrings are really pretty hard-core when you think about it: someone had to punch an actual hole in an area really close to your skull in order for you to wear them. If that's not badass, I don't know what is.

There's lots of hilarious vintage advice out there about wearing earrings that makes breathless, sweeping exclamations like "Larger earrings make the nose look smaller!" and "Avoid drop earrings if you have a long face or short neck!" These ridiculous statements are dated for a reason, because there isn't an accessory that has more of an effect on your face than a pair of earrings—but the style you choose to wear doesn't really matter. Almost any pair of earrings can work for you (no matter what your facial shape), as it's a universal truth that absolutely everyone looks good with a little bit of sparkle, color, and movement by their face. (The actors I've dressed who are reading this are nodding their heads in agreement, because they've all heard some version of this spiel from me a thousand times and they've seen with their own eyes the difference it can make to their look.)

FOUR DIFFERENT WAYS TO WEAR THE SAME OLD EARRINGS

Nobody needs actual instructions on how to wear earrings, but it's really easy to get into a rut and never try anything new. If you're bored of everything you own, try one of these styles on for size:

PEARLS: Natural pearls occur when an irritant of some sort mysteriously gets inside an oyster, causing layers of nacre (the organic matter inside a shell) to form around it as a defense mechanism, resulting in a smooth, round, pearly ball. Cultured pearls occur in the exact same way; the only difference is that the irritant was placed there by a human hand. Both natural and cultured pearls are technically *real*, but since it can take thousands of oysters to get enough natural pearls to make a necklace, most better pearls for sale are actually cultured. Pearls have received a bad rap for being too stuffy and uptight, but whether real or faux, a pair of milky white (or even blush or pale pink) pearl earrings adds a lustrous glow to the wearer's face. (Yes, even your ten dollar pair from the mall.) To keep pearls from being too prim, pair them with their polar opposite: a bohemian hippie blouse, total rocker look, or men's-style suit jacket.

CHANDELIERS: Made to look like dangling chandelier crystals, these earrings aren't just for fancy occasions—so if you have a pair lying around from a wedding that you never wear anymore, try giving them a spin with the most clichéd outfit of all time: a T-shirt and jeans. This may sound crazy, but why save your sparkles for special occasions? Life is short, so you might as well wear something fancy on a random Wednesday in November. Wearing a pair of chandelier earrings to work or to the grocery store is also a good way to jazz up your face when it's a horribly rushed, throw-your-hair-up-in-a-ponytail kind of day. Statement sparklers will even work in the workplace when paired with a toasty, chunky, turtle-or funnel-neck sweater—as the simplicity of the sweater will allow the earrings to stand out. (Also, when you've got every available bit of skin neatly covered, you can be a bit more coquettish with your earrings without it seeming inappropriate.)

HOOPS: Made of circular metal wire in varying diameters (from delicate ones the size of your pinky finger to insane ones that could go around your calf), hoop earrings are a statement-making, face-framing choice. Their ergonomic circle shape makes them extra-complementary to your jaw and cheekbones, but they can tend take a bit of self-confidence to pull off successfully. Some may think that larger hoop earrings are a bit too much to add to a work look, but the truth is that as long as they don't hang lower than your hair, they function as an accent piece—peeking out as you move around instead of calling all the attention to themselves as they would if your hair were worn up.

STUDS: Due to their small size, stud earrings are like your own little secret. So you can get away with wearing any style, symbol, or color  your heart desires, because most people won't even realize what they're looking at—they'll just take in the glint of shimmer and shine the studs lend to your face. So if you've long thought smaller earrings weren't worth the effort, give them a whirl.

WHEN A PAIR IS NO LONGER A PAIR

If you've lost one earring from a pair, embrace a styling trick employed by hip models and fashion designers alike: just make your- 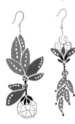 self a new pair using some clever mismatch magic. When done right, a pair of mismatched earrings gives you an offbeat, cool-girl vibe that's hard to beat. It's also intensely practical—because otherwise, you'd be tossing your lonely single earrings into the trash. Here are some interesting combos to try that will have everyone thinking you totally meant to mismatch in the first place.

SHORT + LONG: If you've lost a single hoop, the remaining one is the perfect foil to any single long, dangling earring you may also have lying around. I especially love this look when both earrings are different metal colors.

KEEP IT DIFFERENT—BUT THE SAME: To play it safe, keep your two different earrings in the same metal and stone color family, such as silver with pearls. That small bit of cohesiveness gives you the latitude to go crazy with a mash-up of styles.

EMBRACE THE SILLINESS: It pays to embrace the unexpected. Two slightly dorky, whimsical earrings (like a smiley face and a safety pin) suddenly seem to go together when worn in a cheeky way.

LEAN ON CONTRAST: A delicate, threadlike earring is a great contrast to a stronger, more architectural one. As always, it's all about balance.

COMMON EARRING DRAMAS (AND HOW TO SOLVE THEM)

If you've all but given up wearing earrings because they kill your ears or won't ever stay on, take heart—there are some easy solutions out there to the problems that plague you:

STOP THE DROOP: If your earrings droop, wobble, tilt, or just will not sit upright on your ears, try switching out your regular-style earring backs for ones with a clear disk-and-bullet-style backing. They are available at almost every mall accessory store for a dollar per pair—and will easily provide the extra bit of support and stability your ears need.

GET THE RIGHT BACK: If your earrings keep falling off, it's almost certainly because regular old earring backs (also called friction backs) tend to loosen up over time. Instead, try a fishhook-style earring, since they are way less likely to fall out. Lever-back earrings are also a good option; as the name implies, they have a little lever that keeps the back closed. If you mainly wear stud or post earrings, it's worth investing in a set of locking earring backs, available online or at better jewelry stores. They usually cost between twenty and thirty dollars and will work on 99 percent of the inexpensive earrings you already own. You just push them on when you want to use them (fair warning: it does take a small amount of effort) and squeeze them off to remove. If you're investing in a more expensive pair of earrings, consider asking a jeweler to replace the posts and backs with la poussette locking backs, which work because the back locks itself into place via a small notch located near the end of the earring post. They aren't cheap, but neither is a lost diamond stud.

KEEP THINGS COMFY: If a pair of earrings is turning your ears green, you can buy a special brush-on coating (available online) to act as a barrier between your ears and the offending metal (which is almost certainly made of nickel—since it's the most common metal allergen there is). You can also use clear nail polish to coat the earring posts, but you'll need to apply it (and give it time to dry) before every single wearing, as the protective coating gets eaten away as you wear them. If your ears still turn green even with the nail polish trick, you may need to only wear platinum or surgical steel-post earrings.

WAIT, WHAT ARE THESE FOR?: You know those tiny little pieces of clear rubber that come with some earrings when you buy them in the store? Yes, they are mainly meant to keep the earrings on their backings while they are for sale, but those little backs are also genius at holding in wire or fish-hooked earrings that have a terrible tendency to fall off your ears, especially if you are someone who fiddles with your earrings when nervous or while concentrating. But you can drive yourself absolutely bonkers trying to keep up with those tiny little things, since they are practically invisible and therefore prone to getting lost, so you'll appreciate this news: they are available in a pack of a hundred online for about a buck, so feel free to lose them to your heart's content. They are much cheaper to replace than a lost earring.

BRACELETS: WHY AND HOW

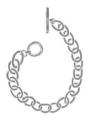

I am a huge fan of the annoying clickety-clack sounds an armful of bracelets makes. It's a way to remind the world that I'm here, I'm taking up space, and I'm noisy, so just deal with it. But I did once have the sound department on a film set approach me with a roll of tape and say, "Can we tape those bracelets to your arm? The clacking is ruining the dialogue on every take!" Whoops.

FOUR DIFFERENT WAYS TO WEAR THE SAME OLD BRACELETS
Adding a bracelet to an outfit can sometimes seem like a bit too much, especially if you work in an office and have to type on a computer frequently. I tend to only wear bracelets on the weekends for this exact reason, but if you still want to wear them while you work, just keep them confined to whichever hand doesn't have to use

a mouse all day long. If you still think you might be a bracelet hater (or feel like bracelets are inherently old-fashioned) try one of these new-fangled styling tricks and get inspired:

BANGLES: Bangles are rigid circles that slip over the hand and onto the wrist. They are best worn in multiples, so mix and match these to your heart's content—metal, plastic, rhinestone, and fabric. It's almost impossible to screw it up, but try staying within a color range to avoid a little kid-style rainbow effect. This means pairing light colors together, dark colors together, or even different shades of the same color together.

CUFF: A cuff is a wide, rigid, open bracelet (usually made of metal) with an opening that allows the wearer to slide it on and off the wrist. Wearing a set of matching (or contrasting) cuffs and no other jewelry at all (aka Wonder Woman–style) is a styling trick that works with almost any outfit to make it look as if you stepped out of a magazine. You'll almost certainly have to adjust the gap of your cuff bracelet a bit upon the first wearing, but keep in mind that most cuffs are only meant to be adjusted about six centimeters from their original size. Carefully bend each end little by little as you put it on to avoid damage—and don't bend the bracelet every single time you put it on, or you will eventually weaken and damage the metal. (Oh, and PS: the gap goes at the inside of your wrist.)

TENNIS: A tennis bracelet features a thin row of bezel-set diamonds or rhinestones and is usually set in either 14k gold or gold-plated metal. The tennis bracelet came into fashion after tennis pro Chris Evert dropped her diamond bracelet on live television at the 1987 U.S. Open tennis tournament and jewelers across the country cashed in. All these years later, I still love the rich old lady chic way a cheap, faux tennis bracelet looks when jumbled up on the same arm as a watch.

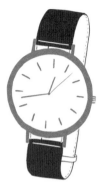

WATCH: It's true: a watch is technically a bracelet. And here's another truth: if you rely solely on looking at your phone to tell what time it is, there's a good chance that some of your pals and coworkers may wind up with the mistaken impression that you are a rude person who can't stop staring at their digital device. Wearing an old-fashioned watch not only solves this problem, it also gives your look an instant boost of gravitas.

MORE, MORE, MORE: WEARING A BRACELET JUMBLE

What the world needs now is not another lesson in how to pull off a jumble of bracelets all worn together at once, but here we are. I want to hate it, but it's an indisputable truth that wearing more than one thing at a time on your wrist is crazy cute. If you want some ideas to make your jumble look a bit more cohesive than if you just put everything on and said, "Oh, to hell with it," read on.

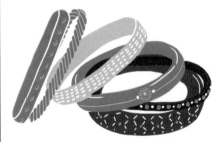

KEEP IT SIMPLE: Keep your bracelet jumble simple by starting with your most practical piece—a watch. This will make the whole look seem easy and thrown together—not forced. Next, add in a piece with a lot of personality, like a statement cuff. Now that you have two bulkier pieces, plug in a delicate chain and two thin bangles to create the perfect five-bracelet stack. And if you're feeling it, you can keep going! The goal is to add depth and interest without adding a ton of bulk.

TRY SOME LEATHER: If you're new to wearing a jumble, try mixing a leather wrap bracelet in with some metal ones. It takes up a good amount of arm space (for a smallish amount of money), making it easy to wear multiple bracelets without adding too much weight—and it's a great way to add depth and color to a boring jumble.

USE A THEME: A good way to start your jumble is by getting a theme going. For example: if you've been collecting Southwestern-inspired bracelets your whole life, pile them all on together, taking care to alternate thin ones with wide ones. And if you love the ocean, chances are you've amassed lots of beachy-themed pieces that should work well when worn all at once.

BABY'S ALL GROWN UP: HOW TO PUT YOUR BRACELET ON BY YOURSELF

A bracelet that has an old-fashioned lobster claw clasp is a nightmare to put on your own wrist. Nothing will remind you that we all truly die alone faster, and I've almost certainly ruined my eyesight by squinting at that tiny little ring like a cross-eyed wombat. In a fit of frustration one day, I used a piece of clear office tape to keep the loop end in place right at the center of the inside of my wrist, which made it a snap to then hook the clasp through it.

RINGS: WHY AND HOW

What's the most famous ring in the world? I think it's a tie between Princess Diana's blue oval-shaped sapphire surrounded by a halo of diamonds (currently living on the finger of Catherine, the Duchess of Cambridge—formerly known as Kate Middleton), and the 33.19-karat Krupp Diamond, given to Elizabeth Taylor by Richard Burton, which she called "my ice skating rink." If you are a person who talks with your hands, consider spending your accessory dollars on unique rings—

since they will help you get your point across with style. An unusual or interesting ring also has the added benefit of making you seem outrageously stylish with just one piece.

FIVE DIFFERENT WAYS TO WEAR THE SAME OLD RINGS

Since they have been manufactured for thousands of consecutive years, the number of ring styles that exist couldn't be cataloged by one, two, or even three books. Regular rings that you've worn a million times don't present any styling challenge at all, but one of these just might.

COCKTAIL: Cocktail rings are a fabulous holdover from the days when muumuus and beehive hairdos ruled. There is only one rule for a cocktail ring: the bigger, the sparklier, the better! If it tends to take over your entire hand, you're doing it right. Crazy cocktail rings are obviously the perfect party conversation starter, but you don't need to limit yourself to wearing them only when the sun goes down. I love wearing a good, gaudy cocktail ring on my pointer finger for a lunch date, shopping, or a ladies' tea—pretty much anywhere I'll be using my hands a lot. Wearing a cocktail ring during the day is also a good intimidation tactic if you know you'll be going over paperwork closely with someone. I've gotten lots of people to agree to things they might not have if I wasn't insistently tapping my behemothly bejeweled finger on a document five inches from their face.

SIGNET: These rings date back at least to the second half of the thirteenth century, when they acted as a small seal, meant as a signature substitute on official documents at a time when few people could write. (This is also why we refer to the closing of a business deal as "sealing the deal.") Historically worn by British royals and flashy, dandy, wheeler-dealer men, signet rings are perfect these days for anyone who wants to inject a bit of classic, faux-aristocratic style to their look. Signet rings are almost always worn on the pinky finger, and are usually built on a thick silver or gold band with a large flat top that has an emblem or symbol stamped into it—anything from a rose to a skull, a family crest, or even a personal monogram. Mixing a menswear-style signet ring with one that is more properly ladylike is a good, subversive styling trick to try, since it takes a bit of confidence to pull off.

MIDI: The rise of the midi ring (one that stops just above your knuckle) means that you can now kind of wear any old ring that doesn't fit your finger properly in a way that screams, "I meant to do that!" But rings intended to be worn around the knuckle are usually thinner than regular ones; otherwise, they could overwhelm your hands and keep you from being able to drive, type, or do dishes. Midi rings always seem a bit outré, because they have the same feeling as one of those statement-making full-finger "armor rings," but they mercifully have none of the movement restriction. They are a good way to tart up your work clothes if you are forced to dress ultra-conservatively on the job, since their delicate yet subversive nature is a nice contrast to a business look. And if you're afraid of losing them, make sure they fit a little bit tight, but not so tight that you can't feel your fingers.

TURQUOISE: A good way to give your boring work clothes a style bump is to add some Native American–style turquoise rings to the mix. The stunning blue-green color of this classic stone adds a warm, earthy feeling to even the most staid wardrobe pieces. Traditional Native American jewelry first popped up in the 1850s as a blend of European metalwork and Native American culture, and prices range from twenty-five dollars for a small ring and well into the thousands for larger vintage ones. When shopping, keep in mind that in the United States, it's illegal for vendors to claim that items are produced by Native Americans if they are not, so it's best to buy from a Native American source whenever possible.

GRANDMA BLING: An older ring passed down from a family member won't look stale or old-fashioned once you pair it with edgier, more modern pieces, and if you start wearing your grandma-style ring every single day on the same hand as your other trendy rings, it'll start to look natural to your eye, no matter what you pair it with.

MORE, MORE, MORE: STACK THOSE RINGS

There aren't any real rules for stacking rings on one finger, but here are some things to keep in mind that will make it seem a lot less strange and intimidating.

TONS OF TEXTURE: Wearing a stack of multiple rings at the same time requires only one thing: lots of texture. Combining simple, smooth items with pieces that have copious amounts of etching, engraving, or raised details elevates a stack from messy to truly fashionable.

REPEAT YOURSELF: Try repeating the same style on each finger— like a handful of different turquoise shapes or various sizes of simple gold bands. You can also play with the idea of wearing one color on your left hand—and another color on your right.

FOOL THE EYE: Wearing three rings of the same width across your index, middle, and ring fingers in a straight line will mimic the way a large, solid ring looks, and it's an easy way to get used to wearing more than one ring at once. (As a bonus, people will think you're wearing brass knuckles at first glance and be way less likely to mess with you.)

MIX IT UP: Varying styles definitely adds more interest. That means interspersing beaded and gemstone rings with simpler bands.

MAKE ONE FINGER THE STAR: If you're going for the super-extra look of stacks on multiple fingers, choose one stack to be your most dominant, eye-catching one, keeping the stacks on your other fingers to a dull roar. Two or three ultrathin rings on the quiet fingers will suffice and keep the whole look from going overboard.

WHAT SIZE RING DO I WEAR?

It's a good idea to figure out the ring size for every finger you might choose to wear a ring on, as knowing your ring sizes will make it easier to shop for inexpensive, interesting rings online. If you don't live near a jeweler who will measure your fingers for you, cut a piece of string or paper and wrap it around each finger—well below your knuckle but not right where your finger meets your hand. Don't pull it so tightly that it cuts off your circulation, and mark (or cut) at the spot where the paper or string meets, then measure the length of your paper or string. Once you have all your numbers in hand, it's easy to calculate your ring size according to the chart below. (Ring sizes also come in half sizes, and those measurements will fall somewhere in between the listed whole sizes. Also, your ring sizes are likely different on each hand since your dominant hand is a little more developed.)

Size 4: 46.7 mm	Size 10: 62.3 mm
Size 5: 49.3 mm	Size 11: 64.5 mm
Size 6: 51.9 mm	Size 12: 67.5 mm
Size 7: 54.5 mm	Size 13: 70.1 mm
Size 8: 57.0 mm	Size 14: 72.3 mm
Size 9: 59.3 mm	

BROOCHES AND PINS: WHY AND HOW

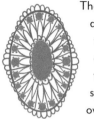

The most bang you can get for your accessory buck is having a small collection of fabulous brooches. Most people think they are a boring, old-fashioned item—so they are usually wildly inexpensive and readily available at thrift and vintage stores everywhere. But with a little clever styling, a sparkly brooch is the most multitasking accessory you can own. (And consider this: those adorable enamel pins made to look like donuts, middle fingers, and dinosaurs that everyone is so bonkers for these days are technically a new-fangled version of the old-school brooch—so feel free to style sparkly, old-lady versions in the same way you would a set of modern pins.)

EIGHT DIFFERENT WAYS TO WEAR THE SAME OLD BROOCHES AND PINS

Keep these styling ideas in mind for the next time you see a cute brooch in a thrift shop and think, "I wish I knew what to do with that!"

PUMP UP A PARTY LOOK: Wear a different jeweled brooch on each of the shoulders or straps of a simple party dress for maximum glam.

WEAR ONE AS A HAIR BAUBLE: Make your own fancy hair doodle in an emergency by slapping a brooch onto a ribbon and wearing it as a headband or as an accoutrement to decorate your ponytail. (I've also made a cute choker or impromptu bracelet out of a wide piece of ribbon and a bejeweled brooch.)

BUMP UP YOUR BEANIE: Add a fancy, sparkling brooch to the front of your dreary winter beanie to elevate it from boring basic and to add a little sparkle by your face on a gray winter day.

EVERYTHING'S BETTER IN PAIRS: Jazz up your winter coat by adding a pair of complementary oversized brooches (like two different floral ones) on each side of your collar.

FANCY FOOTWEAR: If you have a pair of simple fabric shoes (such as Toms or Keds), give them a style boost by pinning a set of mismatched brooches to their tops. I like to use two pins that are different yet related: think a bumblebee brooch paired with a flowered one. (Obviously, this works best with pins that have a flat, straight bar back, since you don't want a stickpin post digging into your foot with every single step.)

TOUGH BUT SWEET: I find that brooches lose some of their staid old-lady vibe when paired with something that is decidedly un-glam, such as an olive-drab military-inspired jacket. The mash-up of sweet and dainty against something tough works like a charm to take off the too-ladylike edge.

DRESS UP A BORING BAG: Adding a sparkly brooch to a daytime bag is a great way to make it multi-task for nighttime activities, too. Just make sure to use one with a locking back so it doesn't fall off easily.

PILE IT ALL ON: Wearing brooches in bunches is the fastest way to make them look modern. Pick one brooch to be your star, then space small-and medium-sized brooches around it in a satellite cluster. I find five brooches to be the max before things start looking too bonkers and overdone.

DON'T RUIN YOUR CLOTHES

To keep brooches and pins from ruining your clothes, choose garments that are sturdier in nature—think denim, cotton canvas, tweed, wool, or corduroy. These materials are not only strong enough to support the weight of the brooches, they can magically erase the holes left behind when you remove 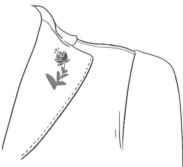 the pin due to the fact that they are thicker, woven fabrics. Delicate, finely spun materials such as silk charmeuse or chiffon will always have a hole in them once punctured—and there's no fix for it.

EXTRA CREDIT: MIX YOUR METALS

If you really want to kick your jewelry look into the stratosphere, consider mixing different metals together. There is actually a bit of an art form to metal mixing—but luckily, it's not hard to master. Metallics are neutrals, and can therefore be mixed and matched any way you like.

The easiest way to start mixing jewelry metals is to find an item that incorporates two different metals to use as your centerpiece—then just add any color metal piece you like to the mix. You can also abide by the 25/75 rule: mix 25 percent of one metal color in your outfit with 75 percent of another. And remember: the hardware on your purse counts as part of your percentages, too! If I'm wearing shoes with silver metal accents and a purse with gold metal bits on it, I like to wear one silver ring and one gold ring to tie it all together. With time (and a little experimentation), you'll start to see how easy it is to mix up your metals like a pro.

BE YOUR OWN JEWELER

My biggest costume design secret is that I'm constantly cannibalizing existing items and repurposing them into something new, personal, unique, and cool. All those random bits and bobs collecting dust in your jewelry box can be revamped into something fresh and interesting with a little cleverness, elbow grease, and a handful of helpful tools.

SPRAY PAINT: A chipped or dull statement necklace, ring, or bracelet can take on new life when you give the whole thing a mono-chromatic coat of high-shine, lacquer-coat spray paint—I'm talking gemstones, chain, and all. Painting gives an ancient piece a fun, candy-coated vibe. Use a bit of matching nail polish to get into all the nooks and crannies if needed.

JEWELRY PLIERS: If a pendant or clasp has fallen off a chain or earring post, don't toss it in the trash! Just buy yourself a small pair of fine-nosed micro pliers, also known as jewelry pliers. You can use them to pry open any jump ring (the small metal ring with a cut in it that holds charms onto necklaces, bracelets, and earrings), reattach it, and push it closed again with your pliers. You can also just use your thumb and a pair of tweezers, but a pair of dedicated jewelry pliers is well worth the cost and are readily available at any craft store for under ten bucks. If your jump ring is lost, bent, or unusable, you can buy new ones by the dozen for about a dollar at your favorite craft store, too. With a pair of jewelry pliers and a handful of jump rings, you can even unleash your inner jeweler by adding charms and pendants to existing necklaces and bracelets in any design you see fit.

GLUE: If your inexpensive rhinestone bauble has lost a stone, just fire up the hot glue gun and stick it back in. A little glue goes a long way, so don't overdo it. (Also, hot glue really is hot! Mind your p's and q's so you don't get burned.) If it's a finer, more delicate piece (such as a vintage item), you're better off using a very strong adhesive glue like E6000 to reset the loose stone. It cures harder and holds longer than hot glue—and is more resistant to water and moisture. (The secret to using an adhesive like E6000 without making a huge mess and having lots of drips while working is to squeeze a glob of it into a bottle cap or onto a piece of tinfoil, then using a toothpick to carefully scoop up a bit and press it exactly where it's needed.)

RIBBON: If your necklace is too short, you can make your own cute extension by pulling off the existing clasp with your trusty jewelry pliers. Then, cut a decorative ribbon in half—and tie one strip to each end of the necklace. You can now tie it in a bow at the back of your neck, adjusting the length any way you want.

GIVE CLIP-ONS A NEW LEASE ON LIFE

Pierced earrings weren't all that prevalent until sometime in the 1970s, so you can easily find a ton of clip-on earrings at bargain prices in vintage and thrift stores—it's actually way easier than you'd think to give them a new life as pierced earrings. All you need is five minutes, a pair of wire snips, some epoxy-based glue, and a set of disk-backed earring posts, which are available at almost any craft store in a pack of one dozen for about four bucks.

Start by cutting off the existing clip-on backs with your wire snips, then apply the flat, disk-backed posts to the backs of your clip-on earrings with a dot of epoxy glue or E6000. Let them dry overnight, then use a set of larger, clear plastic disk backs to support the weight of your new earrings while wearing them. (I like to use a toothpick to make sure the glue is spread evenly on the earring post I'm using, but that's really the only additional tool you need.)

CHAMPAGNE JEWELS ON A BEER BUDGET

I'm actually a total disaster with jewelry—I lose things like it's going out of style. My rings are forever getting left on the sink in public bathrooms or dropped in parking lots because I set them on my lap while applying hand lotion behind the wheel. I'm also always removing my necklaces midday, only to stash them in a purse that I then accidentally donate to a thrift store. I even fail to notice that an earring has suddenly fallen out of my ear until it's way too late to retrace my steps to find it.

I once managed to re-lose a piece of jewelry: I misplaced my class ring immediately after graduation, found it in my parents' garage ten years later, then eventually lost it forever at the beach, which devastated me until I realized you can order a replacement online rather easily. (There was, however, a surcharge to fire up the way-back machine and re-carve a ring using the template of my long-bygone graduation year.) My replacement ring brings me the same pride, joy, and memories as the original, so it was money well spent in my case.

Constantly replacing everything I lose isn't financially sustainable, so I mostly wear a lovingly chosen selection of inexpensive baubles. But on the occasions that I do splurge and buy something real, I always make sure to check out the types of places where you wouldn't expect to find fancy jewelry first. I'm talking pawnshops, thrift stores, charity boutiques, and lower-end department or big-box stores. You'd be shocked at what lurks in the most unlikely of places, all at a deep discount. If there's a jewelry counter to be found at a retail establishment (no matter how crummy it may seem at first glance), you can guarantee I've investigated what it has to offer, often for pennies on the dollar.

Pawnshops in particular are a goldmine of unique, inexpensive items that would otherwise be way unaffordable. I've bought every single pair of real gold earrings I own at pawnshops, including a tiny pair of diamond "A" studs that I paid a hundred dollars for and wear daily. (So, thanks, other A-name person who saw fit to pawn them!)

STOP LOSING YOUR RINGS

To avoid leaving your expensive rings on a bathroom sink, do what my jeweler suggested: Hold the ring in between your front teeth while washing your hands. If you never set it down on the edge of the sink, you can never accidentally leave it behind.

FAKE IT TILL YOU MAKE IT

If you have a lust for better jewelry (but not the budget to match), don't fret—because there are two really clever ways to bridge the gap between the ultracheap chain store stuff and pieces worth thousands of dollars. Knowing what to look for in order to stretch your jewelry dollar further is the key to faking fancy, rich-lady style.

FILLED OR PLATED JEWELRY

A lot of gold jewelry for sale at discount department store counters is actually plated or filled—meaning that other metals (such as rhodium or brass) are mixed in with a small amount of gold to give the look and feel of the real thing (while keeping the price down to a dull roar).

Filled jewelry, in which a layer of precious metal is pressure bonded to the base metal, is more valuable than plated jewelry and is meant to be tarnish resistant. A good piece of gold-filled jewelry does not flake, rub off, or turn colors and most people who have jewelry allergies will find they can wear filled pieces without worry.

Plated jewelry is made of a base metal that has had a thin layer of precious metal brushed on. With repeated wearings, the plating will eventually wear off and need to be redone. Exposure to water, sweat, perfume, makeup, and lotion will hasten the demise of both plated and filled jewelry, so make it a rule not to sleep, shower, or swim in these pieces. Get into the habit of putting on your jewelry only after you've applied your lotion, hairspray, and perfume, since they all contain ingredients that can eat away at it.

It's best to clean plated and filled jewelry with warm water only—using a bit of mild soap when absolutely necessary. If you need to get dirt out of the nooks and crannies of a piece, an occasional light brushing with a new, soft toothbrush is okay—as a used toothbrush will still have traces of toothpaste residue that may be too abrasive and can mar the finish.

A LITTLE GOLD IS GOOD ENOUGH

Almost zero gold jewelry for sale these days is actually 100 percent pure. Gold is far too soft in its natural state, as it tends to bend and scratch easily—making it impractical for everyday wear. To solve this problem, gold is commonly alloyed with different types of metal (such as silver, copper, or nickel) to alter its hardness and color. The gold content of an item is measured in karats: the higher the karats, the higher the amount of pure gold in the piece—and the higher the price.

The bulk of gold jewelry available for sale these days is 14k, but my best el-cheapo jewelry-buying secret is to take a look at pieces made of 10k white or yellow gold. Some may pooh-pooh the idea (I once had a jeweler dismiss it out of hand as "discount gold"), but it actually offers you a pretty great value for the money. It's markedly cheaper than 14k pieces, sometimes almost half the price, and is a great way to have a decently nice piece of jewelry without having to sell a body part.

Ten-karat gold is still almost 42 percent real gold, so as long as you care for it properly, it isn't likely to tarnish or fade in your lifetime. And because it contains less soft, pure gold, it's actually sturdier and harder to bend or ruin than 14k gold. I almost exclusively wear 10k rings because I rap my hands on my desk at work all day long (in both happiness and frustration), and any higher-karat weight always gets bent to bits. Ten-karat yellow gold does look slightly paler than 14k gold, but unless you are a jewelry expert, you won't be able to tell the difference.

IDENTIFYING FOUND OBJECTS

If you've ever wondered whether a ring you found on the ground or at a garage sale was real gold, sterling silver, or diamond, there are a few easy ways to quickly tell what you've found. (Keep in mind that only a jeweler can 100 percent confirm pure gold or silver by using an acid test—but you can buy versions of these tests online and become a pro with a little practice.)

CHECK ANY STAMPS OR MARKINGS: Your first indication that something might not be real precious metal is the lack of a mark. Real gold will have a stamp somewhere that indicates karat (10k, 14k, 18k, 22k, or 24k). Silver will be marked 925, 900, or 800. Sometimes the stamps are crazy small and hard to see with the naked eye, so I use my phone to snap a close-up photo I can then enlarge and study more carefully.

LOOK FOR DISCOLORATION: If the color seems to be wearing off anywhere and showing a different metal underneath, the item is definitely not real gold or silver—it's likely plated metal.

USE A BLEACH PEN: Silver tarnishes extremely quickly when exposed to a drop of a powerful oxidizing agent such as household bleach. (However, this test will also work on silver-plated items—so don't use it as a final indicator that an item is real sterling silver.)

WHIP OUT A MAGNET: If a suspected "gold" piece pulls toward or sticks to a magnet, it's almost certainly fake. But this test doesn't guarantee that the item you've found is real gold, either. To be absolutely certain, you'll need to perform a traditional acid test, which can be purchased online to determine if jewelry is real. It is quite possible for a gold jewelry item to test as non-gold if it is dirty, so make sure your piece is free from grime, lotion, and perfume before testing.

USE THE BREATH TEST: Diamonds are very efficient heat conductors, so if you breathe heavily on a real one, the fog should disperse immediately. A fake diamond will stay cloudy for a few seconds longer. (This test works best with a clean stone, so give the item in question a good polishing with your shirt beforehand.)

ONLINE HUNTING: EFFECTIVE VINTAGE JEWELRY SEARCH TERMS

If you've got a hankering for jewelry that absolutely nobody else will have, you'll want to look to vintage pieces. Not only will you have something totally unique to you, older costume jewelry is usually better made than most modern pieces available at mall stores. Newer pieces will start to wear, chip, and discolor within a year or two, but vintage pieces (some of which are now thirty-plus years old!) will usually still be going strong. This is partly because many older pieces were plated multiple times, making their coating rock-hard. Multiple coats of plating also means that since the base metal is farther away from the skin, people with allergies to certain metals will find that they can wear vintage pieces without having a reaction.

But pay close attention to photos when shopping for vintage pieces online—and always ask the seller for additional close-up photos of any areas that seem unclear. Just because something is vintage doesn't mean you should settle for worn plating, darkened or cloudy rhinestones, clasps that don't work, or missing stones. Half the battle of shopping for vintage jewelry online is knowing just what to search for, so here are some of my favorite vintage pieces to shop for online:

CLEAR LUCITE: Rings, earrings, bracelets, and necklaces made of clear Lucite (a rock-hard, plastic-like material) were hugely popular in the 1960s, but Lucite was actually first in fashion during the 1930s as a furniture material, when Lucite bed frames and coffee tables were all the rage.

Clear Lucite makes an excellent material for jewelry because it doesn't take up much visual space and is therefore less likely to clutter or overwhelm an outfit. Metal jewelry can sometimes weigh heavily on a look, but the light, airy feeling of wearing see-through plastic easily takes it down a notch.

MEDALLIONS: A medallion is a flat, round pendant that has been sculpted, molded, or stamped with a design, such as an oversized gold coin, jeweled disk, or good fortune token. Usually hanging from a metal chain, medallions were extremely popular from the late 1960s through the mid-1980s, so vintage versions are plentiful and easy to find. Medallions are back in style with a vengeance these days, and you can refine your online search for one easily by adding keywords like gold, hammered, filigree, Roman, amulet, or intaglio—but the most bad-ass medallion necklaces of all are the commemorative pieces that secret societies, marathons, schools, or businesses used to give to their patrons.

My prized jewelry possession is a large gold medallion necklace stamped with Julius Caesar's head that was given to Caesar's Palace casino dealers to commemorate the casino's twenty-fifth anniversary. I begged every dealer in the place to sell me theirs and was denied, only to randomly find one for sale at a flea market years later. To score your own very special medallion necklace, take a deeper dive on the web by adding interesting keywords to the word medallion, like commemorative, Liberty Bell, perfect attendance, or Shriners Club. Any place or thing that interests you has likely had a medallion made to commemorate it. Just be sure to add the word necklace to your medallion search in order to pull up pieces on a chain that are ready for wearing.

SNAKES: Ancient Egyptians saw the snake as representing royalty and deity, and during the Victorian era, it was interpreted as a symbol of everlasting love—an idea that took off when Queen Victoria was engaged to Prince Albert in 1839 and wore a ring in the shape of a golden snake with an emerald-set head. Snake motif jewelry has been popular on and off ever since, so vintage pieces ranging from thousands of dollars to just a few bucks are usually easy to find. I'm partial to the gold mesh snake bracelets that were crazy popular in the 1960s and 1970s as part of the ongoing Egyptian Revival, usually featuring emerald green or ruby red eyes and made by companies like Whiting and Davis, Trifari, Monet, and Lisner.

CARDIGAN CLIPS: Introduced in the 1950s as a way to help hold and secure a cardigan on the wearer's shoulders when they chose to wear it open, cardigan clips are really just a pair of pretty baubles attached to small clips and connected by a short length of chain. Cardigan clips are still cute when worn in the manner originally intended, but I love to use them as a way to temporarily gather extra fabric at the back of a dress or top that is too big, instantly giving it more shape without having to break out a needle and thread. Cardigan clips can also stand in for a necklace when clipped on either side of a collared, button-front shirt.

MATCHED SETS: Whimsical matched jewelry sets (usually consisting of necklace, bracelet, and earrings—and sometimes even a brooch) were hugely popular in the 1950s. Sets featuring bugs, crystal or metal flowers, scarabs, cameos, leaves, wings, or cat's eye stones became an art form that accentuated the feminine ideals of the era—and instantly gave the wearer a put-together look. Modern sets of matched jewelry (such as rhinestone sets meant for brides) can tend to look fussy and uptight, but vintage sets have an innate sense of retro fun to them, making them perfectly wearable now. Wearing a matched set is a great way to give a drab look an instant dash of put-together charm.

WATCHES: A reader once wrote to me all worried that she had outgrown her childhood Mickey Mouse watch and should stop wearing it, fearing it was too babyish. I told her she was way, way wrong—that vintage watches are an incredible way to inject a huge amount of personality to a look, and that she was lucky to have one with such personal history to it. Searches for brands like Seiko, Timex, Fossil, Swatch, or Casio will bring up styles you may remember from your childhood, while using interesting keywords like ring watch, rhinestone watch, military watch, bracelet watch, or cuff watch will bring up a ton of unusual pieces you might not have thought to look for.

CLEAN IT UP

There are all sorts of tips floating around the Internet about how you can use random household items (like ketchup, beer, vodka, and baking soda) to clean your jewelry. But these items also have the potential to do damage to your pieces because of their acidity or abrasiveness, and the truth is, you don't need to bother making a mess with all that junk, since most metal and clear-stoned jewelry (real or otherwise) will do just fine with a little dish soap and water, a light brushing with a soft toothbrush, or even just a brisk rubbing with a soft cloth.

Washing your jewelry works like a charm (even better than those fancy liquid jewelry cleaners your local jeweler sells) and costs close to zero dollars. But for the love of all that is holy, do not wash your jewelry over the kitchen sink unless you want to watch it go right down the drain. Also, avoid submerging any jewelry pieces you think might have glued-on stones in water. Use a slightly damp cloth to rub them clean instead—otherwise, the adhesive will soften up, causing the stones to fall right out.

Take special care when cleaning real pearls—a light rubbing with a soft, damp cloth is best. Submerging pearls in water can cause the silk cord to weaken, fray, and eventually split. The damp cloth method is also the solution to clean jewelry made of wood, clay, or other porous materials, like amber, coral, jade, opal, and turquoise, that should never be dunked in water or chemical cleaning solutions.

Water, soap, or a simple damp rag is best for almost every type of jewelry out there, but if you're attempting to clean something made of sterling silver, do yourself a favor and invest five bucks in a special silver cleaning cloth—it makes short work of tarnish and makes it way easier to get into every nook and cranny.

STORE IT

How you store your jewelry depends on how often you wear it—and how much of it you have. I own a shocking amount of jewelry and baubles, and tend to wear at least a little something every single day, so I like my jewelry stored right where I can see it. This means I use a repurposed dresser with lots of drawers, sorting everything into various trays—silverware trays for necklaces, ice cube trays for earrings, even shoe-box lids for bracelets. That way, everything is right in my line of vision when I open the drawers, which inspires me to wear pieces I might otherwise forget I have. I keep the small amount of "better" jewelry I own in clear plastic hanging jewelry organizers, hidden in between my winter coats, far away from prying eyes just in case my house ever gets broken into.

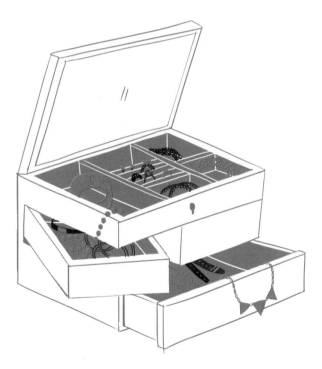

Accessorizing with Eyeglasses

Accessories that live on or near the face draw a ton of attention your way—which presents a special conundrum for those of us who wear eyeglasses. Something that takes up so much facial real estate can make it seem as if there is way too much business going on once you add jewelry to the mix, but just wearing your glasses and nothing else can make your look seem unfinished. The solution to this mess is to make your frames the centerpiece of your look— and add or subtract other accessories until it feels right. Here are some guidelines to follow if you're unsure of how to even begin to pull it off.

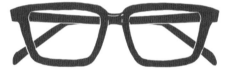

PICK THE RIGHT PAIR

When choosing eyeglasses, it's most important to find a frame that looks good on your face. Don't worry about whether the frames match the idea you may have in your head of what they should look like—just make sure that the shape of the lenses, frame size, and color work for you, because that's the only thing people will notice.

A NECKLACE IS BEST

Necklaces are the easiest piece of jewelry to wear successfully with glasses, because they are far enough away from your glasses so as not to overpower them, yet close enough to your face to add interest.

PLAY WITH SCALE

The key to wearing glasses and jewelry in harmony is making sure there isn't too much of everything happening all at once on your face—and the best way to do so is by paying close attention to scale. If you're wearing a bigger necklace with your glasses, you'll likely want to scale down or skip the earrings altogether, since the earrings in this equation should be the accent, not the main attraction. Achieving proper scale means employing a combination of both size and volume to create a harmonious balance, which means you'll also need to consider how much of a statement your hairstyle is making. If I've just completely confused you, here are three sample glasses, jewelry, and hairdo combos to get your wheels turning:

» Dramatic frames + dramatic earrings + no necklace + hair back

» Chunky glasses + small stud earrings + dainty necklace + loose curls

» Wire frames + thin, dangly earrings + larger necklace + high ponytail

PLAY WITH SHAPE

When choosing jewelry to wear with glasses, the most important thing to consider is the shape of your frames. Your jewelry and frame shapes should be complementary—not identical. For round or circular glasses, stay away from circle-shaped jewelry, since it can tend to create a monotonous, repetitive look. Instead, try pairing round frames with curvy teardrop earrings—or match sharply squared glasses with a pair of squiggly, line-shaped earrings. It might seem like dangling earrings wouldn't play so well with glasses, but they can actually help create space between your eyewear and accessories, resulting in a more balanced look.

PLAY WITH COLOR

Leaning on color to make your glasses and accessories play nicely with each other is an easy cheat. You can go a bit matchy-matchy with a monochromatic color story, such as a pair of dark navy frames worn with cobalt blue earrings—or use a subtle color story, such as light brown frames with a warm, ivory-toned necklace. Brightly colored frames coordinate well with gemstone jewelry, and if you wear frames that complement or match your hair color, you can go a little wilder with your accessories—because since your glasses are blending in with your hair, you can allow your jewelry to pull focus instead.

KNOW WHEN TO SAY WHEN

If you're wearing busily patterned clothing along with your glasses, you may not need to add any accessories to your look—unless it's something that performs a function, like a watch.

KEEP IT BELOW THE BELT

Try focusing your accessory attention to the area well below your glasses. Pick a statement pair of glasses—either something brightly colored or in an unconventional shape—and then pile on the bangles, wear a belt with an eye-catching buckle, and load up your fingers with a few beloved rings. The distance between your face and your arms means you can afford to be bold at both ends—and never have to worry about it looking overdone.

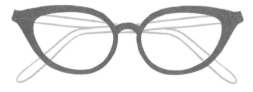

TAKE CARE

Keeping your glasses clean and in tip-top shape is as important as the accessories you wear with them—because if your glasses don't look good, your ensemble won't ever look great. Here are a few easy ways to give your glasses some TLC:

» Cleaning your glasses at least once a day will make your frames and lenses last longer. If you don't want to spring for fancy eyeglass cleaner, a gentle washing with mild soap and water (followed by a careful drying with a soft dish cloth) will keep your glasses spic and span.

» Always rinse your glasses with water before wiping or cleaning them. Tiny particles of dust or dirt are constantly settling on your lenses, so if you wipe those around on a dry lens, you're almost certainly scratching your glasses without even realizing it.

» Never use paper towels, tissues, or napkins to dry your lenses. All of these materials, regardless of how soft they are on your skin, have a textured surface and can easily scratch your lenses. Also, refrain from using the tail of your shirt. If the clothing you're wearing is not 100 percent cotton, the fibers in the fabric will scratch your lenses over time.

» Hair spray, perfume, and makeup can build up on your frames, causing them to get an ugly, cloudy look that can't be removed. That's because it's not simply a buildup of gunk you're seeing, it's the actual finish of the frames being eaten away. Always put your glasses on *after* you've applied your cosmetics and done your hair, and they will last way longer.

» Storing your glasses when you're not wearing them isn't just a great way to keep dust and dirt away from your eyeglasses, it also protects them from getting scratched, bent, or broken.

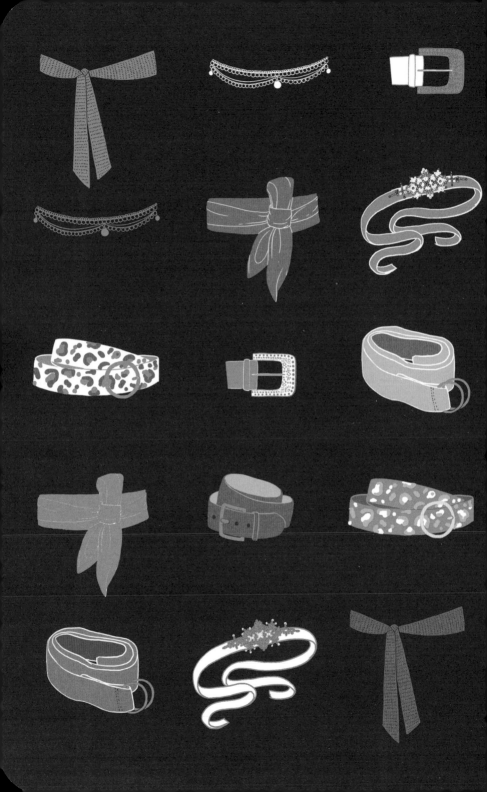

CHAPTER 2

———

HOW DO I BELT?

Here's a style question I get with an alarming amount of frequency: "Hey, Alison, how do I belt?" I always know what the asker means immediately, because while belts can truly make an outfit, they are also cause for much consternation and confusion—and a bad one can really ruin your day by causing you to have to adjust and futz with it constantly. Wearing any kind of belt can be challenging, especially when you're shy about drawing attention to your waistline. And if you've been blessed with bigger hips, sitting down while wearing a waist-defining belt may cause it to instantly force itself upward to your boobs, which is hardly the ideal look for a boss babe trying to run a meeting, get a house loan, or tell some boring dude that, yes, she really is breaking up with him, effective right the hell now.

A BALANCING ACT

To wear a belt successfully, you have to find the perfect combo of belt type, color, and positioning, in addition to pairing it with the correct style of garment. The possible combinations of these factors are endless, so it's almost impossible to give you a one-size-fits-all solution here. But once you figure out the right belt equation for your body, your styling options expand exponentially. When I hold fittings with actors, we try on belt after belt until one clicks—or until we realize that what the outfit in question needs is not actually a belt after all.

If I were to take you shopping, I'd do the same thing to find the right belt for you, experimenting with a million top/dress/belt combinations right there in the store. Sadly, there are very few tried-and-true rules for wearing a belt. But that's not to say you can't eventually get it right—just that it's a game of trial and error. If there was one single truism about belts, it's this: beginning belters will make fewer mistakes if they start out by experimenting with skinnier belts, meaning one inch and under. Thinner belts easily add color, style, and texture to any look, without taking up a ton of space, chewing the scenery, or calling too much attention to themselves.

Sometimes belts are doing very important work, like holding up your pants, but it's also okay for a belt to be worn purely for looks. There's lots of talk out there about belts needing to "defining your waist," but if you are sensitive about drawing attention to your middle, try slinging a belt low around your hips instead. It draws the eye away from the torso and instead highlights your lower half.

A belt is not a miracle worker, but the right one can help nip in a too-big garment, cover up a weird detail, seam, or fabric pucker, or pull together a sloppy ensemble instantly. And if you normally wear more conservative clothing, belts are a good way to go a little wild: think studs, grommets, crazy colors, or prints.

Belts can feel strange when you're not used to wearing them, so give yourself time to get used to the look and feel of extra pressure around your hips or waistline. If you still find belts uncomfortable, look for ones that somehow incorporate elastic. Not only will they stay in place better, you'll also be giddily comfortable all day long.

FIND YOUR BELT SWEET SPOT

The best belt for your particular body is the one that hits your belt sweet spot. Your particular belt sweet spot may be at your natural waistline (which you can find by bending over—wherever your skin folds is your natural waist), or it may be a little higher or lower. The only way to truly figure it out is through experimentation, but here are a few guidelines to get you started on your belting journey:

» If you have an average-sized bust but tend to carry weight around your midriff, wearing a one-inch belt just above your natural waistline is usually the right spot, since the belt will be more likely to stay in place without your tummy causing it to drift upward. A slightly wider (roughly two and a half inches or so) elasticized belt is also a good choice, since it can successfully be worn right over the largest part of your stomach.

» If you're short-waisted and well endowed, positioning your belt a little bit lower than your natural waist will help lengthen your torso. A narrower belt (around one and a half inches) is usually your best choice, since a too-wide belt can tend to take up a lot of room on your already short waist—covering up your midsection and making it look as if your body goes from your boobs straight down to your legs.

» If you have bigger hips, go for a thin belt (about one inch wide) worn right at the smallest part of your waist, since anything wider may tend to ride up mercilessly. The perfect belt for those with bigger hips is actually a metal chain belt, because the weight of it helps to keep the belt down around your waist—instead of letting it float up to your boobs, which can wreak havoc on your entire look.

» Long-waisted peeps are in luck, because they have enough waist real estate to wear any style of belt they please, even extra-wide belts three inches and above. If you are long-waisted, placing your belt a bit above your natural waist is most effective—and can actually help shorten your upper body a tad, making you look more proportional.

THINK ABOUT CONTRAST

Once you've found your belt sweet spot, it's time to decide if you want your belt to blend in—or contrast with your outfit. A low-contrast belt (one close in color to the rest of your ensemble) is usually best for those with waistlines that are short, straight, or otherwise undefined, since it gives the illusion of a long, clean line. Playing around with textured belts (like snakeskin, suede, patent leather, or tweed) while keeping your clothes simple is the best way to add interest to an ensemble without causing a big fuss at your waistline.

A belt that contrasts highly with the rest of your outfit (such as a light pink belt worn with a dark denim dress, or a burgundy belt on a white top) automatically draws attention to your waistline, so if you're going for a more streamlined look, choose a belt that more closely matches the tone of your outfit, such as a hunter green belt worn with a black dress. It will blend in and add a bit of interest without going overboard.

KNOW WHEN TO BELT

Knowing when to add a belt to an outfit (or when to leave well enough alone) is truly an art form. I can't really quantify it in specific terms for everyone, but what I can do is give you a few reasons why anyone would want to wear a belt in the first place. Follow the ones that seem like they'd work for your particular body or style, and you'll have a decent chance of achieving belting success on your first try.

TO CREATE SHAPE: A belt is always the right tool to cinch in an oversized paper-bag waist—or to stop yourself from looking as if you're drowning in a billowy garment. Very body-conscious dresses (such as a bandage dress) already have all the shape they need, so don't bother belting them unless you're going for a highly specific look like a corset belt, which we'll talk about on page 67.

TO HIDE IMPERFECTIONS: A good belt is like a face-lift for your pants, as it can be instantly pressed into service to hide an unsightly detail. If you have a garment with a very visible or totally crooked waist seam that doesn't seem to be doing anything positive for your look, just slap a belt on to hide it. And if your dress has a zipper that bunches up and creates a hump at your back, you can push the hump down and keep the zipper in place with a belt that has some elastic to it. It will act as a "zipper girdle" and keep the zipper from popping up on you all day long.

TO REMIX YOUR LOOK: One of the easiest ways to change the look of an outfit is to add a belt. You'll likely find that adding a belt then inspires you to wear the outfit with different shoes, a different bag, and even different jewelry. For example: a thin, floaty, floral dress you previously wore beltless, with flat sandals and stud earrings, will take on a whole new vibe when you wear it again with a leather belt that has some heft. With the addition of the belt, that same dress suddenly calls out for sneakers or ankle boots, a thin jean jacket, and a bandit-style kerchief—which you'll learn how to tie for yourself on page 83.

TO GIVE THE EYE RELIEF: A belt is the best way to break up a large, boring expanse of fabric that has no interest. Instead of looking like a solid-colored lump, a well-chosen belt creates a focal point for your outfit that gives the eye something to focus on. A belt can also keep a heavily patterned dress from looking like a tapestry filched off the walls of a medieval castle. Case in point: even Scarlett O'Hara had the good sense to add a corded belt to the emerald-green velvet dress she made out of the curtains at Tara.

TO POLISH YOUR LOOK: If you feel like your outfit looks sloppy and you've tried everything to fix it, it's probably worth considering a belt. Many times, a belt is the very thing an ensemble needs for that totally "finished" feeling. If you're wearing a pair of pants with belt loops and a tucked-in shirt in a professional setting, you should most definitely wear a belt—as empty, exposed belt loops can look sloppy and forgetful. And if you really want to polish things off, a gleaming metal buckle in almost any style goes a long way toward making an outfit look smart and put together.

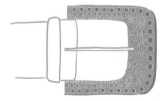

WHAT NOT TO BELT

My accessories mantra will always be "pretty much anything goes"—however, belts are the one accessory that you need to take a little extra care with, because adding a belt to certain garments can go wrong in a hurry. But as long as you avoid belting these five specific pieces, almost anything else is fair game.

T-SHIRTS: I've tried this (both on actors and on myself) and failed numerous times. Maybe it's because of the flimsy fabric—or maybe it's because of the innate casualness of the garment—but slapping a belt over an untucked T-shirt just never seems to work out.

ANYTHING WITH AN EMPIRE WAIST: Not only is belting an empire waist unflattering, it's also distracting and uncomfortable. Nobody needs a belt cinched around their ribs or right under their boobs.

GARMENTS WITH A WAIST DETAIL OR BUTTONS: If the waist of a garment already has buttons or other detailing, just leave it be. You don't want to confuse the eye by layering a belt on top of something already busy with details.

PANTS WITHOUT BELT LOOPS: If your pants rest on your hips and don't have belt loops, you probably won't want to wear a belt. It will almost certainly slip and slide around mercilessly and you'll spend the whole day trying to keep it centered on your waistband.

DRESSES WITH NO WAIST: Belts can add shape and interest to dresses, but using a belt to create a waist in a dress that doesn't have one can result in bunching a lot of fabric together, changing the way the dress drapes and running the risk of looking sloppy.

FIVE ITEMS YOU THOUGHT WERE UN-BELT-ABLE

For every belting "Don't" I could throw at you, there's probably a photo out there of some cutie absolutely killing the same exact style. So you may as well try one of these five combos that seem as if they wouldn't make any sense—and then be as thrilled as I was when I realized that they actually worked.

COCKTAIL DRESS: Belting a cocktail dress is the perfect way to give something you've worn a million times a new look. If you're going to a very proper, fancy event, wearing a thin (about half an inch wide or less) glittery, jeweled, or metallic belt cinched at the natural waist (or the waist seam of your dress, if there is one) is an excellent idea, while a thicker leather belt (around one inch wide) can tone a fancy party dress way down, making it totally dive-bar worthy.

WINTER COAT: If you're tired of your boring old winter coat, try belting it. A one or two-inch belt with texture and dimension (like a faux snake-skin or crocodile print) will give the look a total "I meant to do that!" vibe. This look works best when you know you'll be keeping your coat on for most of the day—that way, you won't have to worry about where to stash the belt once you take your coat off.

FLOWING BLOUSE: A longer silky blouse worn untucked with a low-slung, medium-width belt (between one and two inches) and an A-line skirt is a good way to incorporate shape and structure into a billowing silhouette—while still maintaining maximum comfort.

SHIFT DRESS: A sleek, straight shift dress worn with a medium-width (about two inches max) belt can make this sometimes-boring dress style instantly more interesting. It's best to place the belt directly over any waist seam detail the dress may have, and make sure to avoid any belt over three inches wide—otherwise, it can tend to overwhelm such a straight-up-and-down silhouette.

HIGH-WAISTED JEANS: Yes, you can totally wear a belt with high-waisted jeans, as long as they have belt loops. You'll also have to make sure you can adjust your belt to a shorter length, since high-waisted jeans sit far above your natural waist, where things are likely smaller. A pair of high-waisted jeans also gives you the perfect opportunity to try out a crazily printed or brightly colored belt, like a two-inch zebra-striped or neon-pink number—as bright, fun belts provide great contrast against light, dark, or black high-waisted jeans. Then add your favorite concert T-shirt or ladylike blouse (tucked in, of course) to the mix. It's the perfect way to look polished yet completely casual at the same time.

NEED BELT HELP?
LOOK TO YOUR JEWELS

If you wouldn't wear big, chunky, gold jewelry, then you likely wouldn't wear a belt with a big, chunky, gold belt buckle, either. Taking your belt cues from the jewelry you're naturally drawn to is a good way to never wind up with something you can't quite figure out how to wear.

LIGHT + HEAVY = STYLE

Contrast is what gives a look that extra dash of personality, but it can veer into unfortunate territory quickly—and a poorly-matched belt and shoe combo runs the risk of screaming "sloppy" from all the way across the room. The good news is that if you think in terms of light and heavy, you'll almost never go wrong. For example: if you are wearing a thick suede belt (which is heavy), you'll want to stick to a chunkier, possibly closed-toe shoe (also heavy), such as boots or plat-form sandals. But if you're wearing a razor-thin, Versace-glory-days gold chain belt (which is inherently light), a strappy open-toed heel or bright sandal (also light!) is the perfect match. Alternatively, you can achieve a perfect match by mixing up shades and finishes within the same color family—like a pair of cognac-colored, crocodile-print shoes worn with a dark, chocolate brown ribbon belt.

MATCHY-MATCHY

There's nothing wrong with matching your belt to your shoes and purse, but you certainly don't have to. Matching both will make you look polished and pulled together, but it can also sometimes read as too stuffy or overly conservative. That's not to say you should never do it; just be careful not to wind up looking like Kathleen Turner in *Serial Mom*. But when in doubt (like at a job interview or other formal occasion), it never hurts to lean on matching. A good rule of thumb is that when you are wearing a belt, shoes, and purse at the same time, at least two of them should match. The third item is your wild card and can usually contrast with the rest of your outfit to your heart's content.

THE EIGHT GREAT BELTS

There are a billion belts to be had out there, and it's easy to think you need at least a million of them in order to be stylish, but you really only need a handful to pull off any look you can possibly dream up. The eight belt styles below make up the perfect belt wardrobe—and are what I buy for every actor I ever style.

STURDY LEATHER BELT: The cornerstone of any belt wardrobe is a weighty black or brown leather belt with a simple buckle. It's obviously the perfect piece to pair with a tank top and jeans, but it's also useful when you want to take a fancy dress down a notch.

RIBBON BELT: Whether threaded through belt loops or lazily strung around the waist of a casual summer dress, a ribbon belt is an easy way to add pizzazz to any outfit that a leather belt would be far too heavy for. Florals and watercolor prints work well with a ribbon belt, and as an added bonus, this style is easily adjustable—so it always fits!

METALLIC OR BEJEWELED BELT: A belt with sparkle or a reflective surface instantly gives anything you pair it with a dressier appearance. If you feel like a shiny or bejeweled belt is a bit too bold of a choice for you, try one in the same color family of the garment you are wearing, such as a metallic rose-gold belt with a pale pink dress. And don't be afraid to wear a metallic or gemstone belt for daytime—just consider the rest of your accessories carefully, since something shiny around your waist is already making a pretty big statement.

PATTERNED BELT: Something you wouldn't dare wear in clothing form is perfect to try out as a belt. It's a license to go a bit wild with an animal, floral, or geometric pattern you'd never think you could pull off—because interesting prints and patterns are far less dangerous when deployed in small doses.

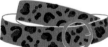

BRAIDED LEATHER BELT: Braided belts are an easy way to add a slightly bohemian (yet still preppy) vibe to any look. Because they're casual, braided belts can also help tone down a too-serious ensemble quickly. I love a braided leather belt paired with something floral, since it takes off just enough saccharine edge, making prints like florals wearable for someone who doesn't want to look too girly.

CHAIN BELT: A chain belt is actual jewelry for your waist, and will instantly become the focus of any outfit, so go easy on additional accessories (specifically oversized necklaces) when wearing one. A wrist cuff or simple earrings are a perfect match here, since they are  far enough away from the belt so as not to compete for visual real estate.

BELT WITH A STATEMENT BUCKLE: Wearing a belt with a statement buckle that sports a classic logo (such as the interlocking Gucci Gs or the name of your favorite band) is a surefire way to make any outfit sing. You can also look for belt straps that have snaps at the end,

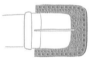 allowing you to mix and match interesting buckles with ease. Once you realize how simple it is to change out buckles and remix your look, you'll find yourself deep in a rabbit hole of interesting belt buckle shopping—because swapping out a plain, boring buckle for one that oozes personality is the fastest, cheapest accessory hack there is.

OBI-STYLE BELT: Obis were originally worn by geishas in Japan to call attention to their curves—and in order to make them look like a present waiting to be unwrapped. Usually made from simple strips of leather or cloth that wind around the waist multiple times, obi belts are widest in the middle (four to five inches in some cases), thinning out to about half an inch toward their ends. This makes them easy to tie any way you like, but they're usually wrapped around the back and then tied in front. My best pal calls obi belts "gut trappers," because they help to keep things firmly in place—and man, she is 100 percent correct.

WHY DON'T YOU TRY: A CORSET BELT

The desire to aggressively accentuate your waist isn't new—images found on ancient pottery in Greece reveal both women and men sporting form-fitting belts adorned with leather rings and straps that constricted and shaped the waist to stop growth. It's safe to say the corset doesn't have the greatest reputation in fashion history, but don't let that stop you from rocking a modern version that doesn't torture your guts at all. Corset belts are all about defining the waist, so I love adding them to an outfit that doesn't have a waist to begin with—like a loose summer dress or oversized shirt.

IF YOU HATE THE WAY A BELT LOOKS, TRY THIS

An excellent styling trick is to layer a longer jacket or cardigan over your belted outfit so that only the front part of your belt peeks out from underneath it. This trick will stop you from worrying about how your belt looks on your waist or at the back by your butt—and will easily add an interesting textural dimension to just the front of your outfit, which was probably where you wanted it, anyway.

A BELT, BUT MAKE IT HOLLYWOOD

For a relaxed, I-could-care-less-what-the-paparazzi-think-of-me look, tuck in only the very front of your shirt—leaving the back and sides of your belt covered. I call this The Hollywood Tuck, and it is best deployed when trying to sneak out of someone's apartment before they wake up. It easily adds just a pop of interest to your outfit and lets the world know that you're wild at heart—but not at all sloppy.

DITCH THE DUMB BELT THAT COMES WITH IT

The belt that comes attached to a dress or top is usually not all that great. There's almost certainly something better out there, and real personal style happens when you bring some of your own flavor to a garment, anyway. Swapping out a belt is very easy—because as long as you replace it with a belt of the same size, whatever you choose should work. That means you can switch out the one-inch braided brown belt on a prairie dress for a one-inch studded leopard number and it will probably still make sense proportion-wise.

YES, A BROWN BELT CAN GO WITH A BLACK DRESS

You'd have to do some fancy footwork to convince me that a brown belt isn't the perfect foil for a black dress—since it adds a sense of lightness that a solid black dress is inherently missing. Just make sure it's a slightly lighter shade of brown (honey brown instead of deep cognac) for maximum contrast, and repeat a spot of brown somewhere else in your outfit, be it a leather cuff, a cardigan, your shoes, or a handbag.

OH BELT, BEHAVE YOURSELF!

The most maddening part of wearing a belt is getting it to stay where you want as you go about your day. If your garment doesn't have proper belt loops (or if your belt is too long and flapping in the breeze), read on for some good solutions to these common problems.

MAKE YOUR OWN BELT LOOPS

If you want to wear a belt with a skirt or pants that lack belt loops, you can easily make your own with two large safety pins. (Just look for a #2 or #3 safety pin, which are one and one-half and two inches long, respectively.) While keeping the head of the safety pin on the inside of your garment, pin it through to the outside of the fabric, threading it back through to the inside of the garment in a wide enough arc to create a de facto belt loop on the outside. (This trick works best with smaller belts, around one inch wide max.) I do this all the time on set when an actor's belt won't stay in place, and because the pin hugs the garment so closely, you can barely tell it's there.

KEEP YOUR BELT FROM FLAPPING AROUND

If the end of your belt is too long (and always flapping around), stick it down with a spot of Topstick men's toupee tape, every costume designer's secret weapon for keeping errant wardrobe items in place. (In a pinch, you can also use regular old double-sided tape from the office supply store.) Just be careful to remove it after every wearing, since it can sometimes damage the finish of a leather or embellished belt. Alternatively, you could make yourself a loop out of a small piece of ribbon to hold the too-long belt end in place. Just tie your ribbon scrap around the width of your belt, leaving a tiny bit of wiggle room to then thread the end of the too-long belt through. In a pinch, you can even make a temporary belt loop out of a very small black hair elastic, like the kind used for braces or to secure the tiny ends of a braid. Simply slide one onto your belt before you put it on, then slip the flapping end under the hair elastic once you've fastened the belt.

CUT IT UP

Sometimes, all you need to do is hack the too-long end of a belt off to solve all your problems, but this may leave an unsightly bare end that reveals the base color of the belt. If it's an inexpensive belt, you can make do by coloring in the bare part with a matching permanent marker, but if it's a pricier belt, you'll want to leave the chopping to a professional. Any shoe repair spot can shorten a belt for you for under twenty bucks.

POKE A HOLE IN IT

Here's the very best advice this book will give you: make the ten dollar investment in a leather hole punch, available at shoe repair shops and online. It will forever change your belt-wearing life for the better. Being able to adjust any belt to work where you want it to on your body is true accessory luxury. You'll have this tool for life, as they are built like a sturdy brick house and won't ever fail you—plus it beats the damaging hammer-and-nail hole-making technique by about a million miles.

ONLINE HUNTING: EFFECTIVE VINTAGE BELT SEARCH TERMS

Before you buy a vintage belt, you'll first need to figure out what size you need. It's never a good idea to trust the stated size on a vintage belt—because not only have sizes changed throughout the years (and sizing wasn't all that standard to begin with), it could also have been altered in a way that makes it smaller than what it's marked as—so always ask the seller to measure the belt for you, starting from where the strap meets the buckle to the very end of the strap. That way, you'll never wind up with an oversized belt meant for a giant—or a too-tiny one that would only fit a child's doll.

SIZING UP A BELT

Measuring a well-fitting belt that you already own is the best way to determine your proper belt size. Lay the belt down on a flat surface, measuring from the tip of the strap to where it meets the buckle. You'll want to round up to the nearest inch here, since you'd obviously rather have your belt a little long than just a little bit too short.

Keep in mind that newer leather belts tend to stretch out over time, and braided belts are especially bad about stretching out, so a belt that fits a bit snug initially will probably wear more comfortably down the road. But vintage belts have likely already stretched all they are going to, so don't count on this trick to get you out of a jam with an older belt that measures just a wee bit too small.

If you don't have a belt you like handy, you can measure your body to see what belt size is best—but first, you'll want to determine where you will be wearing this belt. If it's at your regular waist, measure yourself at your natural waist (which we discussed finding on page 57). If you want your belt to sit below your waist or at your hips, measure around two to three inches below your natural waistline, where low-rise pants would fall. If you're looking for a belt to wear with high-waisted pants, measure about two to three inches above your natural waistline. And take heed: it's important to stand in a relaxed, natural position while measuring; don't push out your belly or suck it in. The measuring tape should be snug, but you should be able to worm a finger or two underneath the tape. Once you've got the right measurement, make sure to add about two inches to allow for proper overlap at the buckle.

Now that we've got all that out of the way, here are some search terms that will likely turn up the vintage belt of your dreams:

CONCHO: During the 1800s, Plains Indians used conchos (round, oval, or rectangular disks engraved with various designs) to decorate horse saddles and bridles. In the early 1900s, their beauty and intricacy led to their adaptation for fashion purposes by Navajo Indians, and the concho belt—consisting of rows of conchos strung along a leather strap or metal chain—was born. Real silver versions from the 1920s and 1930s can run in the thousands of dollars, but inexpensive, non-sterling silver replicas abound online and in vintage stores. To properly wear a concho belt, you have to completely embrace its bohemian nature: think Stevie Nicks at the height of her female rock star power—feathered hair, long scarf, and platform boots.

WOVEN SASH: Sash belts, long strips of woven fabric, usually with tasseled edges, have served both practical and decorative functions in almost every culture for centuries, but colorful versions made in Guatemala (called *fajas*) were intensely popular during the hippie-dippy 1970s. Sash belts are easy to wear because they can be tied either high or low on the waist or hips, making them endlessly customizable. In a pinch, I've even tied one around my head as a headband to hold my hair back. To success-fully wear a sash belt, pair it with something that calls to mind the well-traveled beach bum babe, like a flowy white top, jean shorts, and flat sandals.

FISH SCALE: The best thing to come out of the 1980s (besides *Miami Vice*) was the trend of stretchy elastic belts covered with a multitude of gold metal bits, stacked in an overlapping fashion to resemble fish scales. Usually rendered in glam gold tones, fish scale belts almost always feature oversized buckles decorated with crazy things like lion heads—so it's a lot of look packed into one accessory! Sadly, elastic does tend to degrade with age and get worn out, so ask a few extra questions of the seller before you take the plunge. Once you've scored one, use your fish scale belt to cinch in a slinky disco dress or top off a pair of high-waisted slacks for maximum *Studio 54* glamour.

WESTERN TOOLED: Tooled leather belts (usually decorated with flowers, leaves, swirls, and scrolls) came into fashion during the Wild West era, when guns became too heavy (and dangerous) to simply stuff into the waistband of one's pants. In the 1950s, adding your name to the back of a tooled belt became a trendy practice—and if you search long enough, you just might find a vintage one with your name (or the name of a pet or other loved one) already stamped on the back. Originally championed by country and western singers from Dolly Parton to Tanya Tucker, the tooled belt is a forever classic that can add as much or as little cowboy flair to an ensemble as you want. Pair it with almost any denim item and you've already hit the cowboy note—but mix it with a geometric-print skirt and you've made it completely modern.

MACRAMÉ: Macramé (the art of knotting thread and yarn to create decorative fringe) is believed to have originated in the thirteenth century as an Arab weaving technique, but it exploded into popular fashion during the 1970s in the form of intricately woven belts. A vintage macramé belt is an easy, inexpensive way to add a casual yet worldly edge to a more modern look. Take a styling cue from none other than the king of rock and roll, Elvis Presley, who wore a series of macramé belts in cream, blue, red, and even purple with his jumpsuits during the 1970s (likely for their light, comfortable, non-restrictive nature), and pair a vintage macramé belt with your favorite modern romper.

STUDDED: Studded belts have been steadily popular since the 1960s, so endless versions are available today, both online and in vintage stores—and some of the oldest ones you'll find manage to still look shockingly current. It's a classic style that has been short-hand for punk rock since the time of club CBGB in New York City, and the list of performers who've worn them is endless—from Sid Vicious to Kelly Clarkson. Versions with a single row of studs are thin enough to be threaded through most belt loops, but two-row versions are sometimes a bit too wide for pants with smallish loops. Strangely, I find that wide, three and four-row studded belts are actually easiest to wear, since you can sling them low on your hips over a blouson tunic-style top and add a little bit of punk rock edge to your look without coming off as cartoonish. Just keep your other accessories to a dull roar when wearing such a scenery-chewing piece; a simple pair of earrings or killer eyeglasses will suffice.

STORE IT

Belts are rascally little things, constantly falling down and making a mess no matter how you decide to store them. They can't be easily corralled in a way that also makes them easily accessible at all times—but after years spent organizing actors' closets on the shows I design, I think I've found a few of the best, least expensive ways to get (and keep!) them under control.

GRAB A GIANT CARABINER: Carabiners are large metal shackles (made from steel or aluminum) that have a spring-loaded clasp, which makes opening and closing them a breeze. Commonly used by climbers, boaters, window cleaners, and acrobats, an extra-large carabiner (around eight inches in diameter) clipped over a closet rod makes the perfect easy-on, easy-off ring to store belts on.

SNAG SOME SHOWER CURTAIN RINGS: If you're looking for the ultimate cheap and cheerful belt storage solution, look no further than a set of flexible plastic shower curtain rings from the dollar store—the kind with a small slit to slip them on and off the shower rod. Looping them onto your closet rail means you can store a single belt on each hook, so you don't have to shuffle a bunch on and off a larger ring in order to access the one you want to wear. To save space (and make your belts even easier to look at), slide the shower rings onto a hanger that has a sturdy cross bar instead—I like to use those tubular plastic monstrosities you likely had in college.

INVEST IN AN S-HOOK: You might be familiar with smaller S-hooks meant for hanging up pots and pans in the kitchen, but jumbo-sized versions (around ten inches wide) that hang over a closet rail are the costume designer's gold standard for storing actors' belts in a neat, orderly fashion. Take the time to hang each belt by a large safety pin placed through the buckle, and it will make getting them on and off a breeze. They are available for about nine bucks at everyone's favorite online merchant that starts with an A and is also the name of a rainforest in Brazil.

REPURPOSE A CLEAR PLASTIC SHOE ORGANIZER: Most belts can be safely hung by their buckles, but ones made of cloth, ribbon, or other delicate materials obviously need a little extra TLC. The best way to store these belts is to tuck them into the clear plastic pockets of an over-the-door shoe organizer. Not only are they protected from dust and dirt (in addition to the sagging that can result from hanging), they are also easy to see—and therefore easier to get inspired by while getting dressed.

Color Theory

One of the big secrets to unlocking great accessory style is learning to use color like an artist, stylist, or designer does. Figuring out how an accessory makes sense with the rest of your outfit can seem impossible, but all you really need to make it work is a little bit of color theory—and that means learning to use a color wheel. It's not as hard as it sounds, because a color wheel follows the natural order of color that we were taught about in school: red, orange, yellow, green, blue, indigo, and violet.

You can use the color wheel successfully to style any accessory, from hats and shoes to bags and jewelry, even belts and scarves. But you'll notice that certain colors, such as black, white, gray, and beige, are not part of the color wheel. That's because they are considered neutrals, and you can usually mix touches of them into any outfit successfully. (And as you already know, blue denim matches absolutely everything.) Take a look at some sample color stories below, then jump in your closet and start styling your accessories in ways you might not ever have dreamed of. But take it from a pro: very bright, overly saturated colors are extremely hard to mix and match successfully. Start your color adventure with dusty, muted, or pastel tones, and you'll have way more color-mixing success.

THE COMPLEMENTARY COLOR COMBO

Complementary colors are high-contrast hues that appear directly opposite each other on the color wheel, such as violet and yellow or blue and orange. They only seem crazy on paper—once you get them on your bod, they achieve a visually-appealing combination. Try wearing a pale yellow shirt with a lavender necklace and you'll start to see what I mean.

KEEP IT ANALOGOUS

Analogous colors are those that lie side by side on the color wheel, such as red and orange or blue and green. They make for a bold, outrageously interesting color story, but it's not as hard to pull off as it seems. Try carrying a red bag with an orange jacket (starting with a subdued shade of both until you get the hang of it) and you might wind up surprised at how much you like it.

MONOCHROMATIC MAGIC

A monochromatic color scheme utilizes various shades of the same color to create a pulled-together look that has a bit of variety but is also easy on the eye. Wear a blush-hued beanie, bubblegum pink blazer, and champagne pink T-shirt together, and you'll have nailed this color story perfectly.

THREE COLORS: THE COSTUME DESIGNER'S SECRET

If you want an easy, fuss-free way to pull an outfit together, consider using the three-color rule, one of my best costume-design secrets. Wearing only two colors can be boring, and a four-color outfit can quickly start to get visually overwhelming. That's not to say that excellent, interesting outfits can't be built around two or four colors, but wearing three colors is the ultimate sweet spot that will never steer you wrong.

I stole this idea from the Rule of Three writing principle, which states that introducing characters or events in sets of three makes for funnier and more effective storytelling—and also ensures that the reader or viewer will be more likely to remember what you are trying to tell them. Once I became a costume designer and started dressing people for a living, I realized that the reason the Rule of Three works in both fashion and writing alike is because three things tend to form a pattern, and our brains are wired to automatically understand this formula—so the person viewing your outfit doesn't have to do as much mental work to figure it out.

You don't have to do it all the time, but dressing in three colors can really help when you are in doubt about how to put an outfit together. As you experiment, remember that since black, white, and gray are technically neutral shades, you can mix touches of them in (sparingly, of course) with your three existing outfit colors without causing any fuss. (Anchoring a three-color outfit with a touch of neutrals is also a good way to wear lots of color without it overwhelming your eyes.) This all sounds complicated, but when you break down the science behind it, things become much simpler. A three-color ensemble consists of the following:

A PRIMARY COLOR: This is the main color of your outfit, and will take up most of the real estate on your body. It sets the tone for your whole outfit.

A SECONDARY COLOR: The second most-used color on your outfit, this works as the backup to your primary color. The secondary color's main job is to provide a nice amount of contrast to your primary color.

AN ACCENT COLOR: This color is meant to be used only sparingly— and should work to add some "pop" to the first two colors. If you want to repeat a color in a three-color outfit, it should be your primary or secondary color—never your accent color. Your accent color is special, and a little goes a long way.

Below are some examples of simple three-color outfits that will kick your look into the style stratosphere, but caveat emptor: you'll need to play around with shades and tones before you get the equation just right:

» Olive drab jacket (your primary color), dark purple shorts (your secondary color), burnt orange newsboy cap (your accent color). Plug in a simple white T-shirt to simplify things and you're good to go.

» Medium-blue top (your primary color), burgundy pants (your secondary color), blush pink belt (your accent color). Repeat your secondary color (the burgundy) with your shoes to keep most of your outfit's interest on top.

» Mint green coat (your primary color), candy pink handbag (your secondary color), camel-colored shoes (your accent color). Mix in a pale gray sweater to allow your coat, bag, and shoes to be the star of this look.

» Blue blazer (your primary color), red pants (your secondary color), yellow handbag (your accent color). Add in a blue, red, and black-striped sweater that repeats your primary and secondary colors (the blue and red) while bordering and grounding them with a pair of black shoes.

» Magenta dress (your primary color), royal blue sandals (your secondary color), orange handbag (your accent color). Mix in some jewelry in your favorite metal tone to add a bit of shine, since these colors are already doing a lot of heavy lifting.

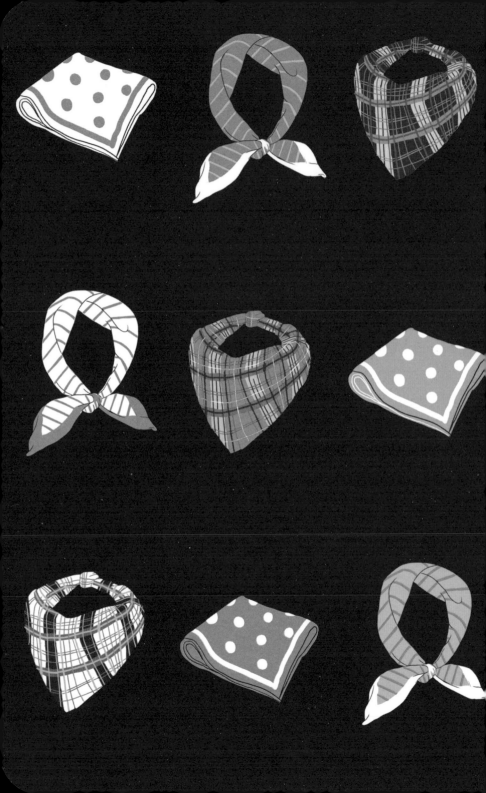

CHAPTER 3

THE ONLY SCARF ADVICE YOU'LL EVER NEED

Figuring out how to wear a scarf in that cute, jaunty way (both emotionally AND literally) without looking as if you are choking, drowning, or impersonating a flight attendant from the 1960s is no small feat. You probably already own (or perhaps inherited) a bunch of scarves that you don't know how to wear, yet don't want to get rid of. Don't feel too bad about it, though, because before I learned how to wear one successfully, I was always Googling things like "What are scarves good for?" and "Why are scarves so dumb?" Once you know what to do with them, scarves are a godsend that can make any lame-o getup instantly better—or add a bit of flair that elevates your outfit from ho-hum to truly stylish. But if you've never learned how to cleverly wear a scarf, it's hard to feel good in one. Did you catch the important word in that sentence? It's *learn*. Rome wasn't built in a day, and you can't just pop out of the womb knowing how to wear a scarf with sass.

THE FOUR-SCARF WARDROBE

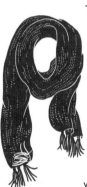

To accomplish almost every single scarf-tying technique there is, you only need to own a few of them: some simple squares and a long rectangle. Square scarves are the ultimate classic, worn by everyone from Hollywood starlets to English royalty. As the name implies, they are perfect squares, ranging in size from extra-small (a sixteen-inch square, often referred to as a neckerchief) to extra-large (a sixty-inch square, often called a sarong). Rectangle scarves are one long piece of fabric, and lengths vary from forty to eighty inches, with widths from ten to fifty inches. A good, workable scarf wardrobe would consist of these four pieces:

» Cotton bandanna, approximately a twenty-two-inch square

» Medium silky square, around a twenty-five-inch square

» Large silky square, about a thirty-one-inch square

» Long silky rectangle, roughly ten inches wide by seventy inches long

THIRTEEN WAYS TO SPORT A SCARF

Part of the reason wearing a scarf seems so confusing is that nobody needs fifty convoluted ways to do it; they simply need a baker's dozen of road-tested styling options to lean on when bad hair days or boring outfits strike. And since absolutely no one has actually wrapped their hair up with a scarf in order to protect a shampoo-and-set from a top-down convertible since 1965, the key to making scarves work for you is to wear them in a modern, relaxed way that packs a punch of practicality.

THE PONYTAIL PUMP: Tying a small scarf or bandanna (either a sixteen or twenty-two-inch square) around a messy bun or ponytail is a quick, cute way to jazz up lazy or dirty hair or to add volume to a scraggly, sagging ponytail. Women with thin hair can use an even smaller scarf (like a men's pocket square) to achieve the same look.

Once you've tied your hair up in a ponytail or bun, fold your scarf into a triangle on the diagonal, and then into a thin rectangle lengthways. Wind the folded scarf around your ponytail or bun and tie it into a knot, tucking a bit of the scarf edges underneath your hair elastic to keep it from slipping off. If you have a big enough scarf (more like a twenty-five-inch square), you can probably even tie the ends into a tidy bow. The great thing about this particular scarf-styling trick is that it corrals all the interest at the back of your head, so it's way less likely to overwhelm your face or clash with your outfit. And a scarf swirled around your ponytail looks good with any outfit because ponytails themselves go with everything!

THE OUTLAW: This look is best accomplished with a bandanna (around twenty-two inches square) that is well aged, rendering it soft and pliable. To tie your bandanna outlaw-style, just fold the scarf or bandanna into a triangle and tie the ends loosely, then pull it over your head and fluff it around your neck until it hangs the way you want.

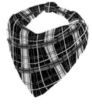

This style works well with a casual button-front shirt, T-shirt, or safari-style dress, but you can also use this technique with a pretty silky scarf, adding a bit of outlaw edge to a ladylike blouse or conservative work outfit. It also helps to protect the delicate skin on your chest from sun damage and keeps prying eyes from being able to look down your top. Plus, if you suddenly find yourself somewhere that smells rank, you've got a handy face mask right around your neck. (Tying superfluous bits of fabric onto my body under the guise of usefulness is one of my favorite pastimes.)

If you haven't had success wearing a bandanna this way, it's likely because it was too stiff to lie nicely against your body. If your bandannas are brand new and way too crunchy, try what we do on set to make new things look old in a jiffy: get a box of real trisodium phosphate powder (called TSP), a degreaser used to prep walls for painting, from your local hardware or paint store. (But beware: don't use a TSP substitute, as it lacks the phosphates you need to break down the stiffness of a new bandanna.) Add one cup to a bucket of hot (not boiling) water, and let the bandanna soak for an hour or so, stirring it every so often to agitate it. Rinse your bandanna well and toss it in the dryer. It may take a few rounds of soaking, rinsing, and drying, but you'll eventually succeed in removing all the stiff fabric sizing from your bandanna—making it perfectly pliable to tie any way you like.

THE CLASSIC HEADBAND: Whether you're dressing for a major home renovation or a casual night out with friends, using a scarf as a headband is both practical and adorable. (It also works well to hide those bangs you are constantly in the process of growing out.) To achieve it, use a twenty-two-inch bandanna or twenty-five-inch silky scarf and fold it into a long rectangle, placing the middle of the folded scarf at the nape of your neck, then tie the ends together on the top of your head. If you have extra fabric flopping around, go for a double knot—it's an easy way to add volume and height to your look, particularly if you have a long face.

Keeping a headband-style scarf firmly in place on your head can be almost impossible—and if you have slippery hair or a big head, I can guarantee you'll spend all day adjusting it. Even locking it in place with a ton of bobby pins doesn't always work, as your scarf will still worm its way out of their clutches and pop right off your head. (Plus, bobby pins are tedious to fiddle with and can be unsightly.) Instead, slip an elastic headband (the kind with a gummy, grippy, lining) over your head , then tie your scarf over it. You can match the headband to your scarf, but it's easier to just use one that blends in with your hair color. Tie the scarf on your head as you normally would, tucking the edges underneath the grippy headband all around. That scarf isn't going anywhere now—no matter how much dancing or head banging you subject it to.

THE OBI BELT: You can easily fashion your own classic obi-style belt (as discussed on page 66) at home with an extra-long rectangle scarf. The exact length of scarf you'll need depends on your waist measurement, but you'll definitely want one longer than seventy inches. For starters, fold the scarf in half so it is about five to eight inches wide. Place the center of the scarf in front of you at your true waist, then wrap both ends around the back of your waist, crossing them over each other and bringing them to the front to be tied.

THE FLIGHT ATTENDANT: It takes about thirty seconds to achieve this scarf style, which works best with a small, twenty-two-inch scarf or bandanna. Just fold or twist it into a thin little rectangle and tie it around your neck using a simple knot. Tilting the knot to the side is the most classic way to wear it, but it also looks cute when the knot is directly at the front of your throat. I also like to spin it around so the knot is at the back of my neck for a sleeker, more streamlined look. This style can help balance things out while wearing something bare, like a slouchy, off-the-shoulder top—as it works to break up a large expanse of skin.

THE TURBAN: A turban-tied scarf is perfect for days when your hair looks terrible (and also on days when your hair looks *really* terrible). It's a lifesaver when you are invited to a party at the very last minute, because you can be out the door in twenty minutes by simply copying Liz Taylor's most classic look during her marriage to, well, just about everyone.

To turn a regular old scarf into a turban, you'll first want to do a little something with your hair, even though most of it will be covered up. If you want all of your hair hidden underneath, take the time to pin your hair flat to your head. (I like to section and roll mine into multiple little "cinnamon buns," pinning them down firmly with regular old bobby pins.) If you want to keep a bit of your hair showing, gather it in a low ponytail at the nape of your neck to keep it from sliding forward and getting in your way. (This is also the time to decide if you want to pull a little bit of your bangs forward to peek out of the turban at the end—if so, don't scrape them back with the rest of your hair.)

Once you're ready to get tying, fold a large scarf (around thirty inches square) into a triangle. Place the tip of the triangle on the top of your head like a widow's peak, then pull it down towards your hairline, letting it hang down over your eyebrows a bit. (You definitely want the scarf to be tilted a bit forward as you tie—otherwise, it can wind up pitched too far back on your head. It will be easy to scooch it back and adjust how you want once you are done tying.) Next, pick up the "wings" of the scarf that are hanging down by your ears and cross them over your face, almost as if you were placing a blindfold on yourself. Twist, don't tie them into a "knot" by your eyebrows, then pull them behind your head and knot them for real. (This knot is what will secure the whole turban, so tie it nice and tight.) Now, all that's left to do is tuck any excess fabric that is still hanging in front of your face up and under the edges, tilt the whole thing back to where you want it to sit on your forehead, and arrange any bits of hair you want to have artfully peeking out. You can also add a jeweled brooch on the front or side to jazz things up, but I like to just add a pair of hoop earrings to balance out all that volume on the top of my head.

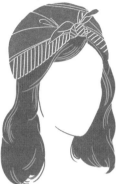

I realize this turban-tying technique sounds convoluted, but it's actually almost impossible to screw this style up. Practice (and patience) will teach you what works best for your particular head. It's a good idea to try your hand at tying a turban when you have some downtime—that way, when you're faced with a hair emergency, you already have the technique mastered.

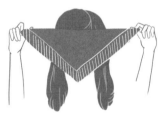

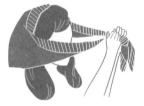

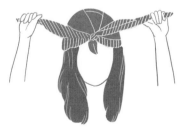

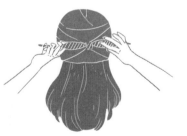

THE BOY SCOUT: If you want to add volume to sloping shoulders (or cover up bare ones, handily turning a sundress into an office-approved ensemble), fold a larger (around thirty-one inches square) scarf into a triangle; then drape it around your neck so the triangle is hanging down your back. Tie the ends loosely around your neck, letting it fall gracefully around your shoulders.

THE BEADED NECKLACE: There's no need to fold or roll your scarf before you start this one: just take a large, thirty-one-inch scarf (the thinner the better), and tie a neat, yet not too-tight knot right in the middle. Then, tie another knot every two inches or so on either side of your initial knot, working your way out to the ends of the scarf. Once you're done, tie the ends together to form a circle big enough to pull over your head.

This will create a lovely beaded effect, which is perfect if you love the look of a necklace but hate the weight and feel of an actual necklace bearing down on your neck and getting tangled up in your hair. Having a scarf stored right around your neck will also come in handy if you suddenly want to put your hair up or cover your face from an onslaught of dust at a music festival. I fervently wish I'd had a clever scarf necklace around my neck when I accidentally laid my head down in a plate of olive oil at an Italian restaurant one New Year's Eve while trying to make my dining partners laugh. I could easily have tied up my oil-soaked bangs in a neat bow if I'd had a handy scarf on—instead, I counted down the seconds and rang in the new year with my dripping-wet bangs plastered to the side of my face.

THE POUF: If you fall in love with a scarf design but find that it is way too small to tie up properly, use it as a pocket square instead. Simply grab the scarf directly in the center and bunch the fabric into a tidy pouf. You can then tuck it into your blazer pocket either pouf up or tails up—your call.

THE BAG CHARM: If you're looking to show off a statement scarf (but it just doesn't suit your current look), tie it into a bow on your handbag handle instead—or weave the scarf in and out of each individual link on a chain bag for a very Chanel-inspired look. Weaving a scarf through a chain-handled bag also works well for bags that tend to slip off your shoulder, but flip to page 131 for an even better solution to slipping bag straps. Having a scarf tied to your bag also comes in handy when your hair decides to take a dive halfway through the day, since you can just wrap it up in any of the ways listed previously to salvage it.

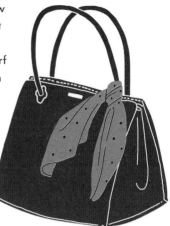

THE PUPPENHEIMER: This one's technically not for humans, but I'm including it anyway—because putting a pet in a bandanna is my very favorite way to style a scarf. To deck your BFF out in style, just fold a small (twenty-two inches square) bandanna or scarf into a triangle and tie it loosely around your pup's neck. If your dog is on the smaller side, you'll need to pick a scarf or bandanna you don't mind sacrificing, as you may need to cut it (the scarf, not the dog) in half on the diagonal so it's not dragging the ground. If you really want to get next level with it, nothing says best friends forever like rocking a bandanna that matches your dog's.

THE SHOULDER SHRUG: Don't spend your money on an expensive evening wrap for a one-night-only fancy event—just use this simple knotting technique to turn medium or large scarves into chic shoulder wraps. First, lay your scarf flat, then fold it in half lengthwise. Next, tie the top left end to the bottom left end in a small knot, repeating the process with the top right end and the bottom right end. This creates two loops on either end of the scarf, and you can then thread your arms through the loops as if you're putting on a shirt.

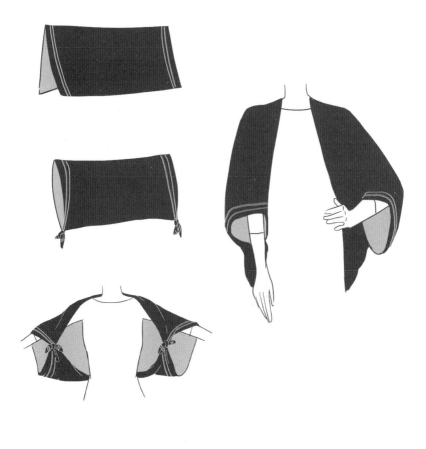

THE EUROPEAN LOOP: In the spring and summer months, a good way to fight an overly air-conditioned office is to tie a light rectangle scarf that doesn't look too wintery into what I like to call the European Loop—if for no other reason than I think it looks très chic and continental. To start, fold your scarf in half lengthwise, creating a loop on one side and leaving both ends dangling loose on the other side. Then, thread both of those loose ends through the loop. You can wear it as tight on your neck as you please, depending on the temperature in your particular ice cube of an office. (Fun fact: Do you know why your office is so dang cold all the time—and why you find yourself sitting at your desk wrapped up like a burrito in an attempt to stay warm when it's actually close to 100 degrees outside? It's because workplace air conditioning temperatures are usually set with the comfort level of dudes in wool business suits in mind.)

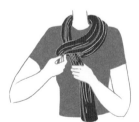
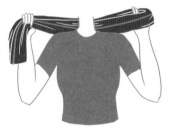
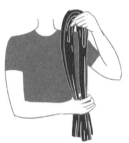
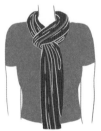

ONLINE HUNTING: EFFECTIVE VINTAGE SCARF SEARCH TERMS

Vintage scarves are almost always a better deal than new ones. Not only are they readily available by the handful in every thrift store in the land, they are usually only about five bucks or less. Most are inexpensive polyester numbers, but if you know what to look for, chances are you'll eventually strike gold and score a real silk one for under twenty bucks—so here are a few noteworthy brands to keep an eye out for on your travels:

VERA: When you think of brightly printed, 1960s-era scarves, you're likely thinking of Vera scarves, designed by the late, great Vera Neumann. Whimsical renderings of animals, landscapes, pop-art florals, and geometric swirls were just a few of her design hallmarks. Vera began designing her scarves around 1947, but the golden age of Vera scarves was from the early 1960s until the mid-1980s, and they are still easily found in vintage and thrift stores today. Look for her cheerful "Vera" signature, sometimes accompanied by her adorable ladybug logo. One caveat: Twenty years after Vera's death, Target marketed a line of Vera-branded scarves, which are still cute but obviously not as collectible as the real vintage deal. Don't pay more than a few bucks for a scarf marked "Vera Neumann for Target" unless you are truly gaga over the pattern.

PUCCI: Italian designer Emilio Pucci was famous for his swirling, kaleidoscopic, geometric prints. He even designed space-age uniforms for Braniff Airlines in 1965, complete with bubble helmets to protect the flight attendants' hairdos. Real Pucci prints are signed somewhere in the design, so give the scarf a good once-over to determine if it's authentic. Pucci prints also typically have very fine black lines separating the colors—with no bleeding onto the colored part of the design. You aren't all that likely to find an actual Pucci scarf languishing in a thrift store, but it's good to know what to look for because the truth is, you never know what you might come across. Some scarves that may appear to be Pucci are actually by French textile designer Jacques Leonard, and will have the name "Leonard" signed in cursive somewhere in the print. Leonard scarves are still collectible, but are not as costly as Pucci ones.

HERMÈS: The undisputed best use of a scarf in accessory history is Grace Kelly repurposing her Hermès one as a sling when she broke her arm in 1956. Not content to be seen around town in a boring old medical device, she immediately pressed her favorite scarf into service instead. Classic Hermès scarves tend toward the larger size (about thirty-five inches square), and you aren't likely to find an authentic one at your local thrift store. But inexpensive reproductions are everywhere, and their equine and astrological themes are as classic today as they were in the mid-1950s.

MADE IN OCCUPIED JAPAN: After World War II, export agreements between the United States and Japan meant that scarves sold in the US had to be marked "Made in Occupied Japan". While this regulation only lasted for about two years, the slow adaptation of production machinery resulted in scarves bearing this mark from about 1946 to 1955. It's an easy way to date a scarf, and since the designs were meant to mimic the popular styles of the era, they are usually vivid, fanciful, and well detailed. "Made in Occupied Japan" scarves have become a bit collectible, but are still relatively easy to find on the cheap.

STORE IT

I'm not exactly saying that the tools you need to store scarves properly are free, but if you happen to work in an office, well, they totally are. Just take a handful of any size binder clip you can manage to scrounge up and use them to clip your scarves onto a hanger. I have one hanger dedicated to my collection of bandannas, one for silky squares, and another for long rectangle ones. This storage system works best on either those paper hangers from the dry cleaner—or on my beloved, slim-line velvet hangers. When stored this way, your scarves take up almost no space on your closet rail, are always close at hand, and are easily visible—instead of stuffed in a dark drawer where you'll inevitably forget to ever wear them.

KNOW WHAT YOU'VE GOT

If you're not sure about the fancy factor of a scarf you've found in a thrift or vintage store, here are two quick things to check for:

» Does it have hand-rolled or hand-stitched edges? This is a huge sign that you are holding a quality scarf. You'll be able to tell because the edges of the scarf will be rolled like a small tube—and will have large, looping stitches holding them down.

» Is it real silk? Most scarves for sale in thrift and vintage stores are made of polyester. But once in a great while, you'll stumble upon a real silk one. Since the labels are often removed from vintage scarves, it's a good idea to spend a little time in a fancy store fondling some real silk ones. It will quickly teach you the difference between polyester and silk, and once you realize what a real silk scarf feels like, you'll be able to easily suss one out in a grimy thrift store and score yourself a real bargain.

Gloves: They're Not Just for Losing

At the 2015 Golden Globes, George Clooney's then-brand-new wife, Amal, caused a giant stir when she chose to wear a pair of pristine, white, elbow-length opera gloves on the red carpet with her black, one-shouldered, Dior haute couture gown. Fashion pundits started Monday morning quarterbacking her look almost immediately: "She looks like she's getting ready to wash dishes!" and "Where is she going, to the prom?" they screeched. A writer from *Vanity Fair* contacted me shortly after the awards for my take on the gloves, which was that Amal probably chose to wear them for two practical reasons: to avoid having to get a manicure, and to hide the wedding ring she'd just snagged from the world's most eligible bachelor from prying eyes.

Elbow-length gloves aren't all that practical for most people's lives, but wearing a pair of short, wrist-length fashion gloves in silk, satin, cotton, mesh, lace, or leather is a next-level accessory-styling trick that instantly elevates an outfit from ho-hum to "Who's that girl?!" It's a practical, yet totally decadent act. When you show up to a party in a pair of gloves in the twenty-first century, everyone thinks you are nuts and comments on them endlessly—but these are both good signs that your outfit has been a roaring success.

Glove-wearing dates back to feudal days (when they were used symboli-cally during the knighting of nobles), but the real golden age of fashion glove wear was from the late 1800s all the way through the 1960s—and for a minute there in 1984 when Michael Jackson rocked a single, spar-kling, Swarovski crystal-encrusted one. Brand new fashion gloves are kind of hard to find, but their crazy-long style reign means that vintage versions are relatively easy to find in every color, pattern, fabric, and style you can imagine. I own a pair of driving gloves (made from perforated leather and featuring a small snap closure at the back of the hand) from the early 1970s that I wear when tooling around Los Angeles, as I'm trying to protect my hands from sun damage as much as possible. At stoplights, people always stare and ask me about them—so if you're into that sort of thing, I highly recommend getting yourself some.

I tend to think that wrist-length fashion gloves look best with garments that show at least a little bit of arm (so people don't think you are wearing them for warmth), but if this book has taught you anything, it's that your mileage may vary—and that every fashion rule was made to be broken. However, there *are* a few classic etiquette guidelines to observe when glove wearing that will hopefully make the whole adventure a bit less confusing.

IT'S OKAY TO LEAVE YOUR GLOVES ON WHEN . . .

» Shopping, in a place of worship, or for outdoor festivities like a garden party.

» Attending a formal indoor occasion such as a reception or ball—or upon arrival at a luncheon or dinner party.

» In a receiving line (unless you're meeting the leader of a country) or while dancing at a formal party.

» At a cocktail party, but just until the drinks and hors d'oeuvres are passed. After that, remove one glove so you can hold your cocktail and snack with ease, then remove them entirely at the dinner table.

WHAT'S MY SIZE?

In order to shop for gloves that actually fit, you'll need to know your glove size. To figure it out, lay your dominant hand down flat, fingers together, with your palm facing upward. Wrap a flexible measuring tape around your palm (just below the knuckles)—but don't include your thumb in the measurement. Your measurement in inches is also your glove size, but I think you should always round up to the nearest half inch or so in order to give yourself a little wiggle room. (The old rule of thumb for men was that your glove size was usually similar to your shoe size, but I've found that isn't always true in real life.)

If you're in between glove sizes, round up for a normal fit or round down for an extra-snug fit. It's also a good idea to always size up a bit for cloth gloves, since they don't have quite the ability to stretch out like leather ones do. If you don't have a cloth tape measure handy, use a piece of string or ribbon, then lay it flat and measure it with a ruler or metal tape measure. If the gloves you have your eye on are sized small, medium, or large, proceed with caution— since the size range could be random. As a general rule, small-sized gloves are a size 6, medium ones a size 7, and large a size 8, but it's never a good idea to trust the marked size of a pair of gloves, so I suggest measuring the gloves themselves around the widest part (much as you did with your hand) in order to determine if they will fit you or not.

GIVE YOUR GLOVES SOME T.L.C.

Like any accessory, gloves need a little tender loving care in order to give you years of faithful service. Follow the rules below and they'll last you almost forever.

» Since leather gloves are usually not waterproof, avoid getting them wet if at all possible. If your leather gloves do become wet, never put them in the dryer or subject them to heat—it's air-drying for those babies only. If even after air-drying, your gloves are a bit stiff, don't worry—the natural oils from your hands will likely soften them again with a small amount of wear.

» Never store your gloves (or any fabric accessory, really) in plastic, since they can't breathe and may start to rot and disintegrate. It's best to store them in your lingerie drawer along with your bras and stockings, or keep them in a cardboard box that lets in a little air (but no light).

» Hand wash and rinse fabric gloves with cool water and the gentlest soap possible, then dry them on a towel, taking care to press them flat into their natural shape (and out of full sunlight to avoid fading). Never, ever put them in the dryer.

OH NO! HOW WILL I TEXT WITH GLOVES ON?

The inability to text with gloves on is part of the beauty of wearing such a throwback look, really—the urge to check your phone is greatly reduced, so you are forced to spend more of your evenings out chatting, dancing, and visiting with friends. It's a form of self-imposed masochism that you may just wind up loving. Most modern gloves have at least one fingertip that's been woven with conductive thread, allowing you to still use your touchscreen phone while wearing them, but you can actually DIY any pair of gloves to make them touchscreen-friendly—just score yourself some silver or stainless steel conductive thread online for about twelve bucks and sew a few discreet stitches of it onto the pointer fingers of your gloves. (Conductive thread is what completes the touch circuit of your screen with your finger.) I like to turn the gloves inside out and stitch through to the front—that way any messy knots are hidden inside, and only a few nice, flat, even stitches are visible when you wear them. Doing this only sounds insane—because it's actually quite easy and really works! (I stitched a little conductive thread onto all my actor's gloves on a period film when they were complaining about having to take their gloves off to use their phones.)

FACE IT: YOU'RE GOING TO EVENTUALLY LOSE YOUR GLOVES

Let me know if you have the secret solution to this age-old problem that doesn't involve some weird series of unsightly clasps, clips, or strings. I've found that balling my gloves up together (like a pair of socks) and always putting them in the same coat pocket when I take them off helps—but still doesn't completely stop me from losing them. If you really want to lessen the chances of dropping a single glove in the snow and slush, keep every costume designer's favorite tool, a large safety pin, in your pocket and pin your gloves together when you take them off and stash them in your pocket or bag. Better yet, just pin them to your coat! It's the grown-up version of those snap clips that keep little kids from losing their mittens.

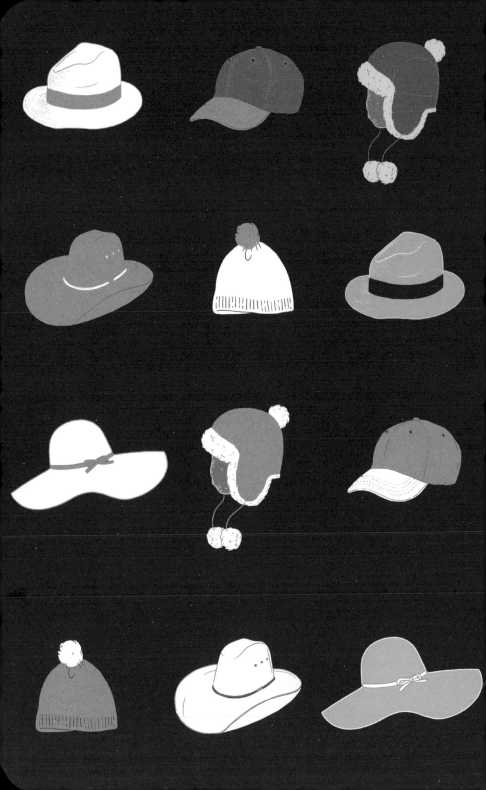

CHAPTER 4

THERE'S A HAT FOR THAT

Anytime a script calls for a character to wear a hat, my first thought is UGH, because so many actors balk at the thought of wearing one. There is no accessory that inspires more fear, loathing, and confusion than a hat. That's because a good one can give you a sense of gravitas that you don't naturally possess, frame your face perfectly, hide some truly horrific hair, and protect you from getting skin cancer—while the wrong one can instantly seem at odds with the rest of your outfit, thereby tanking your entire look. Wearing a hat requires more than a little bit of confidence, and the urge to not even bother trying to find one that looks good on you is understandable.

But there really is a hat out there for everybody, and a ton of cool, useful, interesting ways to wear one—so if you haven't found your hat soul mate yet, don't despair. You just have to try on a lot of them before you find your hat Prince Charming. Eventually one will click for you, and you'll wonder why you spent all that time washing your hair instead of sleeping in and slapping a hat on your mop instead. You don't need to own a plethora of hats, either: once you find what works for you, stick with it. Very few people look good in every single hat style, and if you finally figure out that you look really good in a fedora or a Panama, don't bother wasting any more time trying to make a floppy or bucket hat work.

FACE YOUR FACE SHAPE

Common wisdom says that choosing the right hat is all about finding the correct one for your facial shape, but that's a serious over-simplification. Keeping your facial shape in mind when looking for a hat is useful, but it's not the only way to judge whether a hat will be right for you or not, because I'm here to tell you that there is an exception to every facial-shape rule. However, we all need a place to start, so here are some general face shape guidelines to keep in mind when hat hunting:

OBLONG: If your face is oblong, that means it is longer than it is wide and likely features a rounded chin. Two good hats to try for an oblong face are a wide-brimmed fedora or a newsboy cap, since they both sit a little lower on the forehead and can tend to shorten your face. However, not everyone with an oblong face has a long forehead, so this "rule," of course, is not always true.

DIAMOND: A diamond facial shape is widest at the cheekbones, with a tapered chin and somewhat narrow forehead. Most diamond-shaped faces look great in a classic baseball cap, but hats with a pinched, creased, or indented crown are good, too. As always, there is an exception to every rule, and those with diamond-shaped faces and razor-sharp, model-like cheekbones (those poor, sad creatures!) may find that a creased brim can tend to drag those beautiful, chiseled cheekbones down.

SQUARE: Square faces have strong jawlines, a wide forehead, and wide cheekbones. They can usually pull off floppy hats or hats with lots of curvy lines, such as bowlers and berets. But of course, there's a caveat: A floppy hat can sometimes make a square face seem box-like if your cheekbones aren't quite as wide as your jawline, so you'll need to fiddle around a bit to see what level of floppiness suits you best.

ROUND: A round face is about as wide as it is long, with fuller cheeks, a rounded chin, and a slightly wider forehead. Round faces are usually quite symmetrical and can wear very angular hats with ease, such as a fedora with a slanted brim. This level of contrast is usually perfect, but beware: sometimes the harsh contrast between round and angular shapes can actually over-exaggerate both and look a bit cartoonish.

THE EARS HAVE IT

My biggest hat dilemma is what to do with my ears. I don't have literal elephant ears, but they do cause me a bit of drama when I want to wear a hat—specifically a baseball cap. If I leave them sticking out, I'm kind of self-conscious about them the whole time—but if I tuck them into my cap, they start to throb and hurt within the hour. So before putting on a hat, I've started gathering a small amount of hair from my temple (right in front of my ear) and draping it lightly over the top of my ear. I then secure it to a small amount of the hair right behind my ear with a teeny tiny hair elastic (almost the size of one you'd use for orthodontics). It makes a neat little cover for the tippy tops of my ears, and then when I put my hat on, people only notice my face—not my ears poking out and ruining things.

PARTS IS PARTS

Before you start to try on hats, it pays to know a bit of hat anatomy. Here's a quick breakdown of what we're working with:

» Crown: the top part of a hat that cradles your head.

» Brim: the part of a hat that projects out from the body and wraps around the crown.

» Bill: the front part of a hat that sticks out from the body, covering your eyes; bills are usually found on baseball and newsboy-style caps.

» Crease: the fold or indent in the top of a hat's crown that determines the shape of the hat.

TO START, TRY IT ON RIGHT

If you put a hat on incorrectly when trying it on, you'll never be able see its full potential—and will forever think that particular style of hat doesn't look good on you. You can't just plunk a hat down directly on top (or at the back) of your head, since most hats are designed to be worn tilted ever-so-slightly forward in order to give you a jaunty air.

First, look at the hat to see which way it goes. Usually, the short end of the hat's brim is at the back, but you can also look for the label inside the hat, which is almost always at the back. Once you're sure you've got the hat facing in the right direction, look straight ahead in the mirror without tilting your head forward, and bring the hat up to your forehead. Place the inside front on your brow with one hand, gently pulling the back down with your other hand. (This will make sure your hair stays neatly in place as you position the hat correctly.) While still holding the front brim in place, gently press down on the crown or back brim of the hat with your free hand to secure it in place on your head. It sounds silly, but trying a hat on the right way really does make a difference in how it sits on your head.

DOES IT FIT?

This may seem obvious, but a hat that fits properly will be comfortable. It won't be so loose that the slightest breeze could blow it off, but it also won't be so tight that it squeezes your brow like a vise. A well-fitting hat should touch your forehead without pinching, and the top of your head should graze the inside of the hat's crown, unless you are rocking a baseball cap or Abraham Lincoln stovepipe number. If you find that a hat makes your head sweat or itch, it's likely because the hat you bought is too small; this can cause extra heat and perspiration to build up inside.

HOW TO MAKE ANY HAT FIT

If you find that hats are always too big for your head, buy yourself some hat foam. It is easily available online and usually sold in a roll of twenty feet for five bucks. Hat foam sounds fancy, but is really just self-adhesive foam tape that you cut to fit and stick inside the crown of your hat to pad it out—and stop it from slipping and sliding down on your head. It's what I use on set anytime an actor's hat just won't stay put. If your head is *really* small, consider checking out the hat options available in the kid's department. Not only are they smaller sized, the brims are also shorter and the crowns less tall and pronounced. And best of all, fashion items made for kids these days are usually cuter (and cheaper!) than versions meant for grown ups.

WHAT MAKES A HAT WORTH THE MONEY?

If you're looking to tell a good hat from one of lesser quality, you should take a hard look at how it's made. If a hat is costlier, the material should be relatively soft and somewhat flexible. A well-made hat will also reflect light and color better than a cheap one, making the overall appearance rich and sensuous. For fall and winter hats (usually made from felt, wool, or velour), the material should be soft to the touch, not brittle or scratchy. Spring and summer hats (commonly made from silk, straw, linen, or cotton), should be flexible, not stiff and unwieldy. The brim of a better-made hat will be supple (not cardboard-like), even if it is meant to be rigid. If the hat has a sweatband inside, it should be smoothly sewn, not puckered or rippled. To train yourself to recognize a hat of decent quality, stop into a fancy hat store to take in the details. Once you've seen the real thing, you'll be able to spot nicely made versions out in the wild.

THREE WARM WINTER HATS (AND HOW TO WEAR 'EM)

Wearing a hat in the winter is mostly about staying warm in order to stay alive, but that doesn't mean you have to suffer through wearing something boring that fails to add panache to your entire look. If you need a bit of inspiration, consider one of these styles you may not have thought to try:

WOOL CLOCHE: The classic cloche came into fashion in the early 1900s, and it's still one of the best hats for winter. Not only is wool crazy warm, the downward slope of a cloche's brim makes it far less likely to catch a gust of wind and fly off your head. But in order to keep yourself from looking like an extra from *Downton Abbey*, pair a cloche with a clean, simple neckline and modern accessories only. That means no pearls, no lacy collars, and no overly fussy, frilly, or embellished sweaters. I love a cloche when worn with a classic pea coat and blue jeans.

TRAPPER HAT: Those furry caps with ear flaps that can either be tied up on top of the hat or fastened around the chin to protect your ears from the cold (also known as the hat *Looney Tunes* rabbit hunter Elmer Fudd wears) are called trapper hats, and are usually found on mountain folk in the winter months—but they are actually a great, unexpected hat choice. When something is as plainly warm and useful as a trapper-style hat, it tends to work with whatever you pair it with. But wearing something large and poufy on your head does mean that you'll need to reduce the volume in the rest of your outfit—otherwise, it's just too much material for the eye to take in. Pairing your trapper hat with a chunky sweater and closely fitted leggings will help keep things sleek and streamlined.

BERET: Wearing a beret successfully requires one thing: practice. Whether it's made of felt or knitted with yarn, the beret's floppy nature means it can be shaped and worn in a variety of ways: tilted toward the back of your head with a few poufs of hair pulled out in front, low on your forehead like a beanie, or slanted to the side Frenchie-style with your hair in a braid. Berets that have a self-woven band (instead of the kind with a leather inset band) tend to mold to the head more easily and stay put better as a result. A beret is a great topper for an ultra-ladylike coat and ankle boots, but since a beret is a lot of look to begin with, it's a good idea to choose one that closely matches (or nicely contrasts) a main color in your outfit.

HOW TO WEAR A BEANIE LIKE A COOL GIRL

A beanie is the classic winter choice, but it can be a challenge to wear one in a way that doesn't make you resemble Joe Pesci in *Home Alone*. If you take a quick second to scoot your beanie back a bit to where your forehead and hairline meet, you'll easily achieve that cool-girl slouch. And if your beanie is too tight to properly slouch down on your head, you can gently stretch it out around two or three rolls of paper towels overnight—it will then fit like a charm.

THREE SUMMER SUN HATS
(AND HOW TO WEAR 'EM)

A really good sun hat is usually more than a little dorky. If people are refusing to leave the house with you while you have it on your head, you are probably on the right track, and making your dermatologist very happy. But it is actually possible to avoid sun damage and be stylish at the same time. If you've spent the bulk of your life not wearing a hat in the sun, try one of these three classics on for size.

FLOPPY STRAW HAT: The oversized floppy straw sun hat, with its round top and large brim, is the definitive choice if you want maximum sun protection. No other hat can completely shade your face, neck, décolleté, and shoulders like this one because it's got you totally covered, no matter which way you turn your head or what direction the sun is beating down from. A straw hat looks best with clothes that scream "beach," so wear yours with something light, loose, and airy—like a woven tunic top and shorts. You can also customize an oversized straw hat to match what you're wearing, so decorate to your heart's content with any pins or brooches you have on hand, or just tie a scrap of fancy ribbon around the crown.

BUCKET HAT: The bucket hat (also known as a fisherman's hat) that Gilligan wore on his island is the very same hat made hip by LL Cool J in the mid-1980s when he wore a Kangol-branded version. It is the perfect, practical hat choice if you want something you can crush up and pack in your purse, to be taken out only when needed for sun protection. But its inherent crumpled look means you don't want to pair it with anything too wrinkled or unstructured, lest you start to look a bit like Gilligan himself. A bucket hat takes on a less casual air when you pair it with any shirt that has buttons and a collar.

BASEBALL CAP: This is the heavy hitter of the hat world—a true American classic. No hat has put in more hours keeping sun out of people's eyes, on or off the field. You can get a ball cap that represents any team, product, or idea you can dream up, but for a fresh, unexpected look, try wearing a plain white one. It's the ultimate chameleon, easily matching anything you pair it with, but looks especially fresh when paired with red or royal blue. Oh, and this may be totally obvious, but you'll want to make sure any ball cap you choose for summer is made of cotton, not wool, in order to beat the heat.

HOW TO PROPERLY WASH A BASEBALL CAP

Forget what you've heard about putting your baseball cap on the top rack of the dishwasher to get it clean while washing dishes at the same time. Dishwasher detergents often include bleach (which can discolor your hat), and dishwashers also run at a very high heat, which can shrink and shred a hat. Instead, dunk your ball cap (whether cotton or wool) in a bucket of cool water and a splash of shampoo (which is great for stopping sweat stains in their tracks), letting it soak for twenty to thirty minutes. Then, give any badly stained spots a quick scrub with a washcloth or nail brush. Be careful around stitched patterns and logos, as the stitching can come unraveled if you are too vigorous. Give the hat a good rinse in cool water until it runs clear, then stuff the inside of it with a towel so it will maintain its shape as it dries. Wool hats are notorious for losing their shape after washing, so be especially careful with them.

TAKE IT WITH YOU

Packing your giant straw hat to look glam by the pool on vacation doesn't have to be cause for consternation—because you can keep it from getting crushed and hogging up precious packing space by following this easy hat-packing protocol:

First, pack your heavy items at the bottom of your bag. This includes shoes and thicker stuff like jeans. The goal here is to create a nice flat surface for your straw hat to rest on. Next, take a piece of clothing of decent weight (like a sweatshirt) and roll it up. Place it carefully into the crown of the hat (the place where your head goes), filling the space completely. If there's still room in there, wedge in a T-shirt or pair of socks so the crown is completely stuffed. This will help the hat maintain its shape during travel. Finally, lay your hat upright in your suitcase on the base you built with your heavier stuff. Then, pack the rest of your clothing around the hat, tucking things in carefully so the hat can't move around. If you buy too much stuff on vacation to be able to repeat this process on the way home, just wear your hat on the plane.

CLOTHES FOR HATS

Knowing what to wear with your chosen hat is no small feat—and that's because there is a mix of so many variables going on around your head: the hat color, your hairstyle, jewelry, eyeglasses, and sunglasses. You also have to consider where you're going, what the weather's like, and what sort of activity will be happening when you get there. And if you're anything like me, wearing a hat is a total commitment (my hair doesn't recover easily from being matted down), so if I wear a hat, I'm quite loath to take it off midday. If you aren't sure where to start on your hat-wearing journey, try your hand at some of the ensembles listed below for a bit of inspiration. (As there aren't many day jobs that lend themselves to wearing a hat indoors, I've limited my styling suggestions to off-duty situations only.)

WINTER SHOPPING TRIP

- » Navy blue beanie
- » Amber-tinted sunglasses
- » Mixed-metal bangle bracelets
- » Long winter white cardigan with tie belt or oversized sweater
- » Charcoal gray leggings
- » Black or burgundy combat-style boots

SPRING OUTDOOR EVENT

- » Cream Panama hat
- » Classic aviator sunglasses
- » Multiple thin chain necklaces
- » Tan linen or pale denim button-up shirt
- » Pale blue chino pants or shorts
- » Chestnut flat leather sandals or wedges

SUMMER SPORTING EVENT

- » White baseball cap
- » Wire-rimmed sunglasses
- » Simple gold chain
- » Team shirt
- » Colored denim shorts or jeans
- » Slip-on sneakers

FALL COFFEE DATE
» Forest green beret

» Black cat-eye sunglasses

» Gold or silver hoop earrings

» Brown-toned tweed jacket

» Black round-necked blouse or T-shirt

» Suede knee-high boots

HAT ON? HAT OFF?

Knowing when to take your hat off—or when it's okay to keep it on—is a minefield. Along classic gender lines, the "rules" are that hat styles traditionally worn by men (such as a fedora or panama hat) should always be removed at mealtimes, in houses of worship, at work, in public buildings, or when the national anthem is being played. Fashion hats that have classically been worn by women, such as a fascinator or portrait hat (not unisex-style hats like baseball caps), can be left on at luncheons, weddings, religious services, and even during the playing of the national anthem. But those same fashion hats should generally be removed at work—or anytime they happen to be blocking someone's view.

ONLINE HUNTING: EFFECTIVE VINTAGE HAT SEARCH TERMS

Wearing a vintage hat without feeling awkward requires just one thing: attitude. It also helps to look at vintage photos to see how a particular style was originally worn, then work to create a modern version of that look for yourself. Since they are from a more formal time, a lot of vintage hats are inherently dressy, so they work best for situations or events where one would tend to dress up a bit—such as at an art gallery opening or outdoor wedding. But it really all goes back to attitude, and an easy way to fake an attitude is to work an angle. As Frank Sinatra once said, "Cock your hat—angles are attitudes." He was absolutely right, because sometimes a hat can look ridiculous until you tilt it a bit forward, backwards, or to the side. If the idea of buying and wearing a vintage hat still seems daunting, try some of these search terms for guaranteed success.

PILLBOX: The pillbox hat was made incredibly famous by First Lady of the United States Jacqueline Kennedy. It is a simple, round hat with upright sides, a flat top, and no brim. Since pillbox hats have been in style for multiple decades, they are usually easy to find in vintage and thrift stores. They look fantastic with poufy party dresses—because when your outfit is already akin to a colorful ice cream sundae, why not put a cherry on top? If you are apprehensive about wearing one for the first time, test it out during the winter when at least everyone else is already wearing some sort of hat, too.

NEWSBOY: This is a rounded hat that fits close to the head with a stiff brim in front. Usually made from wool, tweed, or cotton, newsboy caps are a distinctly English invention and were classically worn to school, for casual wear, and with suits. They are a great way to add some tomboy spark to any getup that reads a bit too ladylike, or anytime you feel the need to look more like either Oliver Twist or Brian Johnson, legendary lead singer of AC/DC. Wear one with a button-front shirt and an argyle sweater for a cute weekend look, adding a tweed blazer to the mix if you want a little more polish. It's totally okay if the tweeds on your jacket and your cap aren't an exact match—just keep them in the same color family and you'll be fine. For example: a brown checked tweed hat paired with a brown herringbone tweed jacket will work just fine, while a gray houndstooth tweed jacket wouldn't be such a welcome addition to the mix.

1970S FLOPPY FELT: A floppy felt hat is an easy-to-cop style that adds an instant hippie-tinged finish to any look. And you don't even need to spend your hard-earned money on an overpriced, newer version, because a vintage one is not only less expensive, it's also likely to be better made and far more distinctive. A floppy felt hat in a deep wine or burnt orange shade is the perfect way to dress up a casual outfit—such as a chambray shirt paired with white or black jeans.

STRAW COWBOY: The classic cowboy hat can be a lot of look when you're talking about an old-school heavy felt version, but straw styles (specifically open-weave ones) are light, airy, easy to wear, and totally flattering. A straw cowboy hat is also perfect for protection from the sun and is a great way to toughen up a too-sweet dress.

CLEAN AND DISINFECT BEFORE YOU WEAR

Any vintage hat you buy will need at least a little T.L.C. to make it ready for wear—even if it's just a bit of routine disinfecting before you pop it on your head. To make sure no creepy-crawlies are living on a new-to-you vintage hat, put it in an airtight plastic bag and then pop it in the freezer for about two days. This will kill almost any living organism that could be lingering on the hat, but to be 100 percent certain, leave it in that airtight plastic bag at room temperature for another three days. Living things are aerobic (meaning they need air to remain alive), and this one-two punch should kill anything that has made a home on your hat. But you're not done disinfecting yet! Once you take it out of the bag, give the hat a spray inside the crown with an antibacterial or antimicrobial spray (or even a bit of tea tree oil spray), making sure to get the intended area rather wet with your application. Allow the hat to air-dry, and you're done.

If a vintage hat is visibly dirty, you'll be shocked at the amount of cleanup you can achieve by hitting it with a lint roller. Just make sure you're using the masking tape kind, since velvet ones can tend to grind in dirt and dust. Slightly filthier hats can be cleaned with a soft-bristled hat brush (available for about eight bucks online) to carefully remove any loose dust or dirt. The color of the bristles should be dark for a darker-hued hat and light for a lighter-colored one, and take care to brush gently in a sweeping motion rather than scrubbing, since you don't want to grind in any dirt. Once you're done dry-brushing, lightly dampen a towel (wringing out as much water as possible) and rub the hat in a counterclockwise/circular motion to remove any deeper dirt or dust. If you are using the correct amount of pressure, the hat should not get soaking wet as you clean it. Carefully pat the hat with a dry towel once you're done to make sure any lingering dampness is absorbed.

If a vintage hat has visible stains, you can give them a careful once-over with a lightly dampened dish sponge—just take care to use the soft side, not the abrasive scrubby one. Rub the stain counterclockwise to the grain of the hat, using gentle pressure. The goal is to wipe the stain off—not to aggressively dig it out of the hat. If you're faced with an oily stain, you may be able to draw it out with a generous application of baby powder, baking soda, or cornstarch by liberally sprinkling the powder of your choice on the stain, letting it sit for a few hours, then carefully brushing it off the hat. If you see improvement but the stain is still visible, repeat the process a second time.

If all these stain removal methods have failed, you can try sanding your hat with the finest-grit sandpaper available. But you'll want to be extremely gentle—and only sand the stained area. Don't force the sandpaper into tight spots, and make sure you stop sanding as soon as the stain is removed. It works best on hats made of felt, and you should undertake this fix at your own risk—because the odds of accidentally ruining the hat you're trying to save are high. And a final word of warning: never, ever put any hat (other than a beanie) in the washing machine. It's way too harsh for almost every style of hat. If your hat has gotten that dirty, it's time for a trip to a professional hat cleaner.

THE POWER OF STEAM

If your felt hat has a dent or is otherwise bent out of shape, you may have a little luck coaxing it back into shape using a steady stream of steam. If you bought a hand steamer on my recommendation in my first book, this is the time to break it out! Otherwise, enlist a helper who can direct the steam of an iron toward your hat as you work it gently back into shape. It should go without saying, but I'll say it here anyway: you should never attempt to steam a hat that is on your body—and always wear a pair of dish or gardening gloves to protect your hands from the hot steam—because it will for sure burn you.

STORE IT

The only way to keep a hat from getting dirty, dusty, or beaten up in the depths of your closet is to store it property—and that means keeping it in a classic hatbox. Hatboxes may seem like a throwback, but they are actually readily available in places you might not ever think to look, from big box stores to vintage dealers. You could even use a cardboard box left over from your online purchases—just cover it with some leftover wrapping paper if you want to jazz it up. If you can't manage to scare up any sort of box, wrapping your hat in tissue paper and storing it in a paper grocery bag is a decent alternative. But never, ever stack hats on top of each other—it can cause them to become stretched out, crushed, and misshapen.

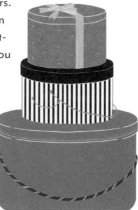

Six Evening Pieces Everyone Should Own

Unless fancy affairs regularly fill your social calendar, you only need a few accessory pieces in your arsenal for any glam event—and then you'll never find yourself sadly carrying your daytime bag to a black-tie event, desperate to stash it under the table as soon as you arrive.

A BAG THAT ISN'T FULL OF CAT FOOD RECEIPTS

Don't cart your work bag stuffed with trash out to a fancy event; instead, carry a small, structured bag in satin or metallic leather (either clutch-style or with a thin strap so it can easily be carried over the arm, freeing up your hands for eating, drinking, shaking hands, or other more nefarious pursuits). But heed this reminder: proper etiquette says you should never stash your evening bag on the dinner table, no matter how beautiful it is. It's on your lap underneath the napkin or on the chair behind you, always. Nothing extra, including your cell phone, is meant to be placed on the table at a proper luncheon or formal dinner. (For even more on bags meant for evenings out, flip ahead to page 126.)

A BORING OLD SHAWL (THAT IS ACTUALLY QUITE USEFUL)

Most evening garments employ a complicated system of straps, beading, and flounce that you couldn't get a coat on over—even if you tried. A simple (or sparkly) woven shawl is the best replacement for a bulky jacket—and looks much more chic tossed over your shoulders if the AC at an event proves to be too much. Jazz it up (and help keep it closed) with one of those fancy brooches you've collected over the years—but never knew what to do with.

HOT SHOES THAT AREN'T FEET KILLERS

Evening shoes don't have to hurt to look good. Flashy flats and glittery low-heeled numbers are where it's really at these days— because nobody looks their best when hobbling around in crippling heels (or even worse, going barefoot when they can no longer stand the pain). Look for flat, T-strap sandals with gems, low booties with openwork or cagelike embellishments, or short-heeled pumps done up in luxe satin fabrics—and don't forget that a pair of simple pumps can be boosted into the fancy-pants stratosphere by adding a set of sparkling vintage clip-on earrings at each toe to act as dazzling shoe clips (see more on page 163.) (For much more on good alternatives to painful high heels, hustle yourself over to page 153.)

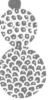

SOME SHOULDER-DUSTING EARRINGS

Shiny, shimmering, shoulder-dusting ear baubles are the best choice to make the most of night-out updos. A pair that mixes rhinestones, pearls, and multiple metal colors will match almost any evening look out there, meaning you'll only ever need to buy one single pair to be set for life.

A SERIOUSLY CRAZY RING

If pierced ears aren't your thing, a selection of bordering-on-gaudy, knuckle-dusting cocktail rings will keep you clinking drinks in style. While I personally think it's hard to go too far with any evening look (because anything sort of goes once the sun sinks), you can always make a pretty big nighttime statement with one single, well-crafted bauble like a giant, sparkling ring.

A SEQUINED SCRUNCHIE

An easy shortcut to flawless nighttime style is keeping a few bejeweled hair baubles on hand. I'm talking combs, clips, bows, barrettes, headbands, hairpins, tiaras, hair sticks, and crowns—even sequined or velvet scrunchies. (Yes, scrunchies are back for good, despite Carrie Bradshaw's screeching about them in *Sex in The City*. There just isn't a better hair holder that is kind to baby-fine hair, doesn't leave dents when you take it out, and gives an immediate height boost to flat, lifeless buns and ponytails.) I've rescued some truly unsalvageable hair right before a big event by just slapping it into a high, perky ponytail topped by a sparkly elastic—but if you find yourself in a pinch without one, it's pretty easy to fashion your own with that fancy brooch you were using to hold your shawl closed earlier. A few bobby pins through the pin back should hold it tight—no matter how much dancing and drinking you subject it to.

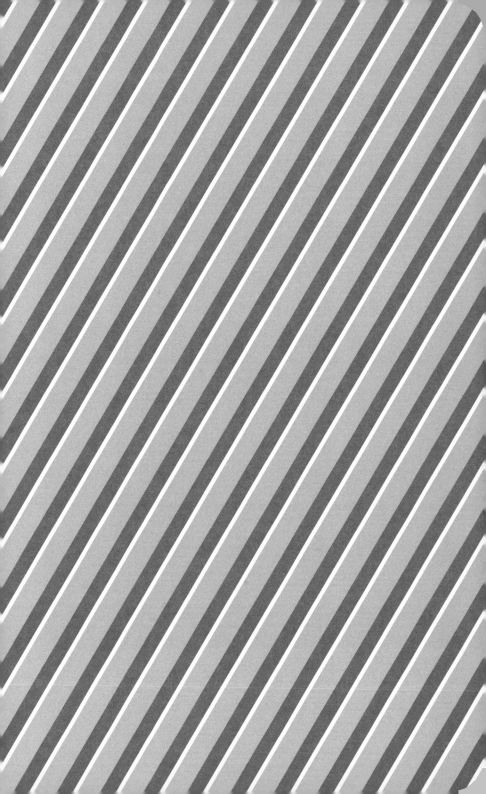

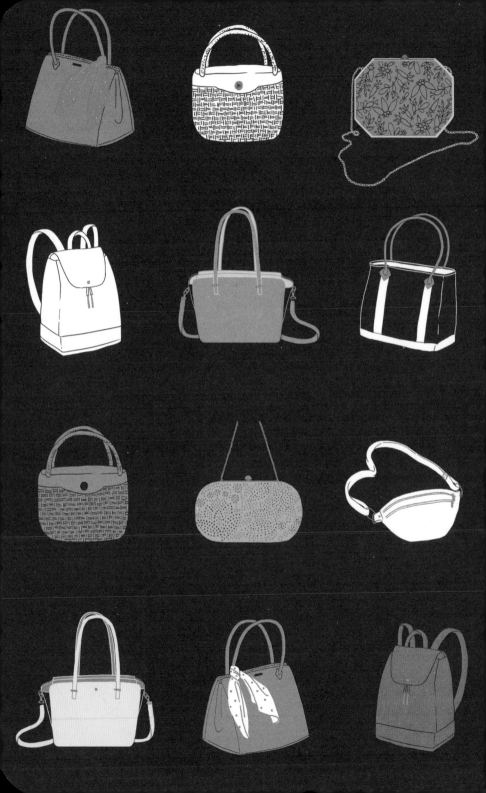

CHAPTER 5

THE PURSE UNIVERSE

If a purse is just a glorified pouch to carry your crap around in, then why did I recently stumble upon an online message board that was filled with people taking photos of their handbags riding shotgun in the passenger seat of their cars? There were thirty-nine pages of these photos to be exact, and they were like glamour shots in a photographer's portfolio, with the bag's straps arranged as artfully as if they were a model's graceful limbs. Careful attention was paid to lighting, background, and composition.

Even though they are intensely practical, purses hold a lot of sex appeal— since they secret away our most intimate possessions. The old adage that one should never poke uninvited into someone's handbag still holds true, and the tantalizing question of what someone could possibly have hidden in their purse will clearly never die. How else can you explain the endless popularity of those "What's in Your Purse?" features in magazines and the games at baby showers where attendees are quizzed and given prizes for producing all sorts of inane, random items from their handbags? Having an arsenal of strange things at the ready in your handbag not-so-subtly signals that you are a smart, prepared, with it, and totally together individual. Whenever I'm at a party and someone needs a nail file, bobby pin, wet wipe, or flashlight, I pride myself on being the one to have it at the ready in my purse.

The main reason purses exist in the first place is that women have long been forced to tolerate clothing with woefully inadequate pockets. Women didn't even carry bags for the bulk of history—garments in medieval times were heavy enough that pockets sewn into the seams could carry everything they needed. In the eighteenth century, dresses had detachable pockets worn inside petticoats that were easily accessed by slits in the dresses themselves. But the winds of fashion always change, and by the nineteenth century, clothes had way less space to fit pockets—so it became fashionable for women to carry tiny bags called reticules. By the early twentieth century, garments became even lighter and thinner, meaning pockets went almost completely by the wayside. Those tiny reticules of the nineteenth century grew into something larger by necessity, and that's how we wound up in the modern purse era: we were conned.

I truly believe I could run for office on a platform that promises "A Pocket on Every Dress," because those who choose to wear men's clothing instead of women's are happily stuffing their necessities into a plethora of pockets—seven or eight alone exist on every single men's suit. As long as clothes marketed to women lack adequate pockets, they will be forced to spend money on purses. That's because it's quite convenient to have a place to shove your wallet, keys, phone, medicine, tissues, hand lotion, lip balm, battery charger, and any purchases you might make throughout a day. I'm not saying that clothing manufacturers are specifically part of an elaborate system designed to oppress women, but if the purse fits, carry it. I'm somewhat mollified by the fact that modern life demands so much gear that more and more men are now forced to carry a bag of some sort everywhere they go, too. Civilization clearly needs pockets to exist, so until we get the pockets we so richly deserve, we're all going to be stuck carrying some sort of purse.

CAN ONE BAG RULE THEM ALL?

You don't need to have a different handbag for every outfit you ever wear, but carrying the same purse for all occasions just doesn't work. People are forever asking me to find them a handbag they can carry twenty-four-seven, and they're always disappointed when I reply that there is no such thing. A giant leather work tote will weigh down a casual Saturday sundress, while a light, summery bag with wicker details will look out of place with a heavy coat in the dead of winter. You'll also find that your everyday bag tends to detract from your outfit if you carry it to a fancy wedding or cocktail party. So to get through life, you'll need a small—yet mighty—collection of at least three basic handbags that can take you wherever you need to go with style.

THE DAILY DRIVER: Your main bag should be a large, sturdy bag in a dark color. Think a doctor's-style bag in rich chocolate brown, an over-the-shoulder saddlebag in a deep wine color, or a simple black top-handled satchel. This should be a practical, attractive bag that looks as at home on your daily commute as it does at a casual dinner, and the straps should be generous enough to spread out the weight so it doesn't cut into your shoulders. In an ideal world, you'd have two main bags—one that goes with black and cool tones, and another for brown and warm tones. If your budget won't stretch to accommodate both, determine which shade dominates your wardrobe—and spend a bit more money on that one, because you'll be putting it through the wringer with hard, daily use. You can then pick up an inexpensive bag in your secondary color, since it won't be getting quite as much road time.

THE CASUAL BAG: Your second bag should be a medium-sized, lighter-weight bag (like a canvas or nylon number) in a neutral shade that is your go-to for days off and weekends. You want something that won't weigh you down—but will still fit all your necessities. Light tan, cognac, olive drab, or navy blue are great color choices for a secondary bag that can go with any casual ensemble.

LIVE A LITTLE: Your third bag—a phone, wallet, keys, and lipstick-only-sized number for nights out or special occasions—is where you can really go wild, since it presents an excellent opportunity to add some eccentricity to your look. Don't worry too much about choosing a top-quality special-occasion bag, because you won't be carrying it every single day. Don't be afraid to try something outside of your usual style, like a bag that's bedazzled, studded, or covered with feathers. The zanier the better, and not to worry—because it's so small, it won't overwhelm your outfit no matter how crazy it is.

IF YOU HATE PURSES

Being a purse hater means that you're constantly losing stuff and kind of always look as if you're just making a quick run to the store. If you dislike carrying a purse (but still need to have some of your possessions with you while you're out and about), why not try one of these alternative methods of carrying your junk around instead?

FANNY PACK: If the term fanny pack conjures up the image of a tiny old lady sitting at a slot machine chain-smoking, you may need to update your reference. These 1980s middle school accessories have made quite the comeback—for no other reason than that they are incredibly practical and useful. Fashion is nothing if it only looks pretty; it needs to serve the user, too. But you don't need to settle for a boring nylon throwback—instead, look for a sleek, structured, leather one with a longer belt that can also cinch in an oversized top if needed. Just keep in mind that a fanny pack (called a bum bag in the UK) isn't meant to be worn over your actual fanny or directly in front of your stomach either. Kick yours over to the side of your hip and you'll never risk looking like a Florida retiree living it up at Disney World.

TOTE BAG: The lowly tote bag can seem like a total throwaway item until you decide to use one as a replacement for a regular handbag. Tote bags are an excellent purse alternative, as they are light, don't pull focus from your outfit, and come in handy when you hit the grocery store on the way home. Carrying a cotton tote instead of a purse is also a great way to let people know what you're into: NPR, farmers' markets, clean beaches, or The Smiths.

CROSS BODY BAG: A cross body bag is the perfect choice for a rock show, day of shopping, or any place you need to spend money with two hands. Having your necessities close at hand without being saddled by a huge shoulder bag is incredibly freeing. However, let's be real: a cross body bag doesn't look all that great on anyone with a large chest, since the strap can tend to bisect your breasts mercilessly. But, honestly, not everything you wear has to always be the most flattering thing ever. Sometimes practicality and ease trump a perfect appearance. Still, those with larger boobs should try carrying a cross body bag that has a wider strap—and wear it directly in front on your stomach rather than on your hip. This hack will help spread the weight of the bag over a larger surface area, resulting in it digging in between your boobs far less.

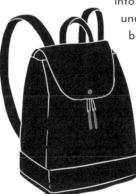

BACKPACK: If you ever decide to switch out your giant tote or purse for a backpack, you'll quickly realize that regular old bags dig into your shoulders and make the weight uneven on each side of your body—but a backpack allows for equal weight distribution, making it the most comfortable bag you've ever carried. Find one made of leather or wool (with statement zippers and hardware) and you'll probably toss your regular work bag out for good.

YOUR PHONE IS AN ACCESSORY

Chances are you spend a lot of time with your phone in full view of others—whether it's on the table at dinner (which is so very bad and rude; please agree to stop doing this and I will, too), in front of you while waiting for your morning coffee, or peeking out of the back pocket of your jeans. So why not treat it like an accessory and kit yourself out with a small wardrobe of different phone cases? I've got a basic protective case that I use when I'm busy on set, a brightly colored one with donuts and aliens all over it for weekend use, a metal-edged designer version for upscale events, and one with onboard lighting for when I know I'll be taking photos with all my friends. The small amount of effort it takes to switch out my phone case based on what I'm wearing (and where I happen to be headed) is well worth it—since it transforms a perfunctory item into a fun accessory.

TERRIBLE, HORRIBLE, NO GOOD, VERY BAD BAG DETAILS TO LOOK OUT FOR

All bags are not created equal—and spending more money doesn't always guarantee you will get one of good quality. When considering the bag you want to be your daily driver, keep an eye out for these telltale signs that a bag may not be of a good enough quality to justify the price.

TOO MANY POINTLESS POCKETS OR COMPARTMENTS

A ton of pockets may seem like a good idea for organization, but pockets that aren't big enough serve no purpose—and compartments that are too big mean your stuff will likely disappear into them forever. If you've ever reached deep into the interior pocket of a bag you haven't carried in years and found your favorite expensive lipstick that you thought you'd lost forever, you're picking up on what I'm putting down here.

A BAG THAT IS ALREADY TOO HEAVY

Carrying a too-heavy handbag practically guarantees you'll wind up with terrible shoulder and back pain. Try setting your current handbag on a scale to see what it weighs—and prepare to be shocked at how much junk you are likely carrying around. Before you buy any bag, pay attention to what it weighs while empty—and curate what you cart around with you carefully to avoid needless, pain-inducing weight.

POORLY DESIGNED STRAPS

Make sure the straps aren't too long or too short for your body. Avoid bags with straps that are pencil thin—they'll cut into your shoulders mercilessly. This is sadly too true of the chain-strap bags I love so much—I don't even consider buying them anymore unless they have a padded leather bit underneath where the chain rests on my shoulder. Double chain straps are markedly better, since they distribute the bag's weight more evenly across your shoulder—and I have had some success getting my shoe repair genius to remodel a few really pricey bags with a little leather cushion on the straps in order to lighten the load.

BAD LINING

Take a close look at the bag's interior lining. It shouldn't seem poorly sewn or flimsy. The items you carry can quickly manage to worm a hole through crummy, badly sewn seams—and then you'll find yourself forever having to fish your lip gloss out of the space between your bag's lining and its outer casing.

WHY WON'T MY PURSE STAY ON MY SHOULDER?

If you've been suffering through life with your purse constantly slipping and sliding off your shoulder (a common problem with bags that feature too-wide straps or straps made of fabric and slick leather), take heart: the problem isn't your shoulder, it's that the designers of most purses haven't bothered to give a minute's thought to making the bag's straps ergonomic and suitable for the human body to carry for long periods of time. Special shoulder strap pads exist, but the fastest way to stop slippage is to cut up one of those clear, self-adhesive gel pads meant for making shoes fit better, and then stick it on the underside of the offending purse strap. They grip like crazy, and your purse strap won't be able to slide off your shoulder even if it wanted to. Just be sure you want it there for good since it could remove the coating on certain types of bonded or artificial leather if you remove the adhesive.

BETTER BAG DETAILS

The idea of buying a purse as an "investment piece" is actually kind of bunk. People should be investing in stuff like stocks and bonds—not purses. I love Gucci bags, but I'm under no illusion that they will build me a house someday. All those "cost per wear" scenarios conveniently fail to mention the monetary returns your cash could be reaping if you were to invest it with a good financial planner instead of parking it on your shoulder in the form of an expensive handbag. That's not to say you should never spend a little more on a nicer bag in a style you think you'll love for a long time, but don't be too bowled over by brand names—because simply spending more doesn't always mean you're purchasing an extremely well-made item. Get in the habit of performing this four-point check on any bag you're considering spending beaucoup bucks on—and you'll never find yourself rueing a bad purse purchase ever again.

LOOK AT THE STITCHING
The stitching of a bag should be consistent all over, and there shouldn't be any loose or stray threads. If it's a patterned bag, the print should match up well at the seams.

CHECK OUT THE BAG'S ZIPPERS AND HARDWARE
A big sign of a quality bag is how the zipper opens and closes. It should glide smoothly and freely. Other closures (such as buttons or magnetic clasps) should also open and close easily without sticking or causing you to struggle.

INSPECT THE STRAPS AND HANDLES
The place where a bag's straps or handles meet the bag's body are important, since those areas bear the most intense pressure with daily use. Avoid spending too much money on bags that have glued handles or straps, since they will eventually separate. You want ones that are securely stitched down—otherwise you risk breakage at the guaranteed most inopportune time.

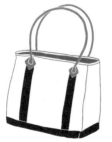

SEEK OUT BAGS WITH SPECIAL DETAILS
A bag that has feet on the bottom means it won't get dirty when you set it down, and a bag with an attached lanyard for your keys will save you from digging in a dark, cavernous hole every time you need to access them.

IS THIS BAG REAL LEATHER?

Simply looking at the label of a bag is a foolproof way to identify if it's made of real leather. If it's real, it will usually proudly say so right on the label. You should also closely examine the finish of any bag you are considering purchasing. Fake leather bags will have pores arranged in a neat, consistent pattern, while real leather will have inconsistently placed pores, since it is made from an actual animal hide. Real leather also has a distinct smell to it, so spend a little time sniffing around in a store that sells fancy leather purses. Become educated on what you're looking for, and you'll never find yourself being taken advantage of.

WHERE THE HELL AM I SUPPOSED TO PUT MY PURSE?

As I was sitting in a restaurant bemoaning the lack of anywhere to put my handbag recently (the chairs had those dreadful rounded backs, there wasn't an extra seat I could steal, and the floor was filthy), I looked around and discovered that every single purse-carrying human in the restaurant had each employed a different method to stash their bags. I sat with mine perched annoyingly on my lap, another person was lucky enough to have a spare chair at the table to rest theirs on, and yet another decided to just say "forget it" and plunked their bag right on the table. The third person held their bag tightly between their legs, resting it on the tops of their feet—while the fourth person kept their bag on their shoulder the entire time they ate. The fifth person just tossed their nylon bag directly on the floor, likely because they knew it was machine washable, so they could deal with it later. (Those of you whose default move is to stash your purse on the floor had better not do one iota of research about how many germs are on the bottom of the average handbag—then multiply that by the square root of dirty restaurants, because you'll die at how disgusting your beloved handbag can get.)

The whole ordeal made me scratch my head and wonder why, after dining out as a species for centuries (or maybe just a hundred years, whatever), have we still not come up with the definitive solution to this dreadful problem? Etiquette books say you should stash your bag behind you at the back of your chair, but that doesn't work too well if the chair is open-backed—and it's crazy uncomfortable to be perched on the edge of your chair for an entire dinner because your handbag is digging into your back.

Very fancy establishments (like the lobby tea at the Peninsula Hotel in Beverly Hills) bring a little pouf to the table for you to set your bag on, and the better ramen joints in Japan all have clever little wire baskets under the table, meant to stash your handbag, jacket, and umbrella while you're eating. Certain drinking establishments have even thoughtfully provided hooks underneath the bar to hang up your purse and coat, but at most restaurants, no thought has been given to this problem, so you're just out of luck.

I canvassed every purse-carrying person I know to brainstorm possible solutions to this pressing problem, only to determine that there isn't really a good one—short of carrying around one of those newfangled purse hooks that uses the law of gravity to balance your purse on the edge of a table. But I can't remember to drag one of those along with me every time I go out to eat—and carrying a bunch of extra junk around with me is not how I'm looking to live my life. I thought about bringing along a plain canvas tote bag to set my purse down on, but again—here's yet another item I have to plan ahead to bring, and I then run the risk of looking like my wacky best pal who always brings a plastic grocery sack to the movies to protect her legs from the filthy seats.

After much careful consideration, I think I've hit upon the best two options available: either never carry any purse you can't wear slung across your body as you eat, or don't be afraid to ask your waiter to bring a spare chair to the table so you can have a place to set down your bag. The latter is what I've started doing, and I've only encountered pushback once, when the waiter told me they actually didn't have a chair to spare—but that he would gladly bring me a high chair that wasn't being used to stash my purse in. I said yes instantly, and the people I was dining with that night still mention it every time I see them.

TRUE LUXURY: CARRYING A DIFFERENT PURSE EVERY DAY

Once you get a decent wardrobe of purses going, you'll find yourself wanting to actually carry them—which means having to transfer all your belongings from one bag to another rather often. But don't waste tons of time switching all your daily necessities from one purse to the other—just compartmentalize everything. A clever system of various-sized pouches from large to small (like a set of Russian nesting dolls) makes swapping bags a breeze and will keep you from having to go on an archaeological dig every time you want to reapply your lipstick.

Plus, keeping your cosmetics corralled in their own water-repellent pouches will keep your handbag looking new longer. Nothing makes the inside of a bag more disgusting than product spillage, and lids are forever mysteriously unscrewing themselves from bottles of lotion in my purse, making a huge, disgusting mess. I have one medium-sized pouch for my cosmetics, a smaller one for gum, tissues, and

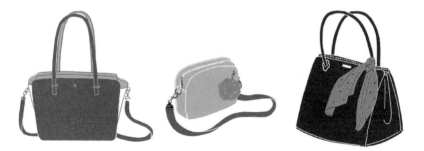

feminine products, a tiny one for my phone charger and head-phones, and another one for my pens and my checkbook. (I actually use various styles of inexpensive zippered pencil cases from the dollar store as my purse-sorting pouches, since they're cheap as can be and are usually translucent enough that I can easily see what's inside.) You can also use a small nylon craft caddy with various-sized pockets from the craft store (available for around ten bucks) to keep your purse contents organized. Just lift it out of one bag and pop it into the other as you race out the door.

DITCH YOUR GLASSES CASE

Don't waste valuable space in your purse with a bulky sunglasses case—instead, pack a bandanna or scarf that you can tie them up in safely when they aren't on your face. As a bonus, you'll then have a scarf handy in case your hair takes a turn for the worse while you go about your day. For all the ways you can make a scarf turn a bad hair or terrible outfit day around, consult page 83.

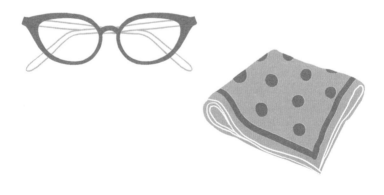

PERFECT PAIRINGS

Matching your purse perfectly to your shoes may be a thing of the past (buying bags and shoes as a set was all the rage in the 1950s), but that doesn't mean you should just throw any old ones on together. Here are some tried-and-true purse and shoe combos that will complement each other and add interest to your entire outfit (without looking as if you played dress-up in your grandmother's closet.)

METALLIC AND MATTE: Pairing a metallic with something matte is a good way to let the metallic piece truly shine. Shimmering silver shoes will work well when paired with a black or deep burgundy bag—while bronze or gold shoes will look great when matched with a warm, rich, chocolate brown purse.

LACE AND SATIN: Pairing two fabrics known for their light, lady-like qualities (such as lace heels with a satin clutch) is an excellent styling trick.

LEOPARD AND RED: Doubling up on patterns can go bonkers fast, so pairing a patterned piece with a solid color that pops is a good way to be bold without taking it too far. A leopard skirt or coat worn with a red shoe is a classic—but you can really substitute any clean, clear jewel tone for the red and be just fine.

PATENT AND VELVET: A smooth leather bag can sometimes look at odds with a sleek patent leather shoe, so play with texture a bit by pairing such a high-shine item with a bag made of rich, plush velvet.

CANVAS AND NYLON: If you're heading to a baseball game or amusement park, you may want to leave your heavy leather bag at home. Canvas sneakers that can be tossed in the wash and an easy-to-clean nylon bag are the perfect choice for an event where a tray of nachos or beer could be poured on you at any moment.

ONLINE HUNTING: EFFECTIVE VINTAGE PURSE SEARCH TERMS

If what you want out of a bag is a dose of originality, your best bet is to shop vintage. Even the hottest "It" bag will probably seem out of date before you can justify or amortize the purchase price, so why not press a lower-priced throwback bag into service rather than spend big bucks on something current? Here are some sample searches to get you started.

TOOLED LEATHER BAG: A tooled leather bag gives you the beauty of an elaborately decorated horse saddle in handbag form. Most tooled bags come in a warm chestnut tone that allows them to easily straddle color lines and match almost anything—and the beauty of a tooled handbag is that you can pair it with pretty much any outfit. It's even a nice foil to very modern styles, since it can warm up a cold look and help take things that are a bit too stuffy down a notch. And you might think a bag this inherently casual wouldn't be proper enough in a work setting, but that's not the case at all. Look for more structured versions with extra-special decorative hardware that make themselves a bit more office-appropriate—and make sure you keep it within the same color family as your belt and shoes in order to look as professional as possible.

MAGAZINE CLUTCH: Made to resemble a rolled-up magazine (and usually made with the shellacked cover of a real vintage one), this hard-sided clutch was popular in the 1970s—but modern versions are still being made today. It's such an interesting piece that it easily turns something as simple as jeans and a bright sweater into a street-style-worthy ensemble.

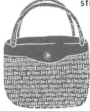

WICKER BAG: Also known as the perfect bag to take on a summer outing, a wicker bag doesn't weigh a hot-weather look down the way a heavy leather bag can. A wicker bag is also good for slobs, because it's easy to clean—so it's almost impossible for it to become stained. You can spill ice cream on it or set it down in the grass to your heart's content, as any mess will wipe right off.

CARPETBAG: These are exactly what they claim to be. Bags made of carpet are an easy way to add a lot of interest, texture, and personality to your look. They were incredibly popular in the 1960s, and a classic vintage brand of the era to keep an eye out for is JT Carpetbags—also known as the California Carpetbagger. A carpet-bag is the fastest way to give an outfit a truly authentic, vintage feel—without wearing actual vintage clothes.

MINAUDIÈRE: A minaudière is a small, hard-shelled bag that is usually made of metal and covered in gems or rhinestones. Also known as a clutch on steroids, the minaudière is meant to be a piece of jewelry all on its own. The story is that Charles Arpels (of legendary jeweler Van Cleef & Arpels) was inspired to invent the minaudière after watching a friend's wife use a metal Lucky Strike box as her handbag for an evening out in the 1920s. A minaudière is incredibly beautiful—but insanely inefficient. Since it is so structured, there is zero leeway to cram extra stuff in one. It is inherently worldly, sophisticated, and mysterious, but only carry one if you foresee a low-maintenance evening on the horizon (meaning you don't need your cell phone, car keys, or lots of extra cosmetics on hand). Winter is the perfect time to rock a minaudière, since you can cheat and stuff anything that won't fit into it in your coat pockets. The most famous (and costly) minaudières are made by legendary purse designer Judith Leiber and come in bejeweled designs and shapes ranging from elephants to Mickey Mouse to cupcakes.

FANCY DESIGNER BRANDS: Certain purse brands can run in the hundreds or even thousands of dollars when purchased from a vintage dealer who knows what's up, but that doesn't mean you can't still accidentally find a gem in a junk or thrift store. If you are a dedicated shopper and know what to keep an eagle eye out for, you'll eventually score something worth major coin for just a few bucks. Here are a couple to know:

» Whiting and Davis: Makers of mesh metal bags consisting of hundreds of small metal tiles fastened together that look like liquid silver or gold, Whiting and Davis purses were especially popular from the 1920s through the 1950s, and they are still made today. Prices for both new and vintage ones should run from sixty-five to one hundred and fifty dollars, depending on size, style, and intricacy.

» Enid Collins: You've almost certainly seen an Enid Collins bag, even if you didn't realize it at the time. These purses (and their many copies) are made of wood or woven linen and feature intricate decorations (usually of bugs, birds, flowers, or other items in nature) done up in rhinestones, sequins, and paint. You can expect to find them priced anywhere from twenty-five to one hundred and fifty dollars. In the late 1960s, kits to "make your own" Enid Collins–style bags were immensely popular. This may surprise you, but when in good condition, these reproduction bags are just as collectible as the real thing.

» Gucci, Valentino, Christian Dior: The licensing frenzy that took place from the 1970s to the 1990s means that some of these vintage logo bags can now be found at an affordable price. That's because they're technically considered to be of lower quality, as they were made by machine and not hand-stitched in Europe, where labor is costly. Usually maxing out in price at around three hundred dollars, most of them still hold up stylistically today. This is a great way to dabble in a little bit of logo mania without breaking the bank—and to never find yourself carrying the same logo bag that everyone else has.

VINTAGE BUYERS BEWARE

In 1948, the US government imposed a huge purchase tax on leather goods, which prompted an instant rise in the production of faux leather. This explains why so many bags from the 1950s were made of imitation leather and plastic materials. Avoid purchasing any that have a sticky or tacky feeling to them, since this almost always means the plastic or faux leather is decomposing—and there is sadly no cure. You can extend a vintage bag's life (and help stave off decomposition) by always stuffing it with tissue or an old T-shirt to help it retain its shape, so the sides don't stick together and further degrade—and by storing it in a cloth bag to prevent it from drying out, since storing plastic in an airtight box stifles airflow—but it's really just a matter of time until all plastic and imitation leather bags eventually meet the same sticky fate.

Vintage leather bags show the most wear at their edges, but can easily be freshened up with some leather dye. I like to use Angelus-brand leather dye, since the quality is unparalleled—plus it comes in endless fashionable colors. Start with a clean, dry bag (you can use either a fancy leather cleaner or a well-wrung-out damp cloth to get it sparkling) and then apply the dye sparingly. Never use the applicator that comes with the dye—it's best to pour some onto a clean, soft cloth instead, since this will allow you to control how light or heavy the application is. Buff the dye in thoroughly, allowing your bag to dry overnight. It should look as good as new by morning. But know this: dyeing a bag will not restore cracking leather—it will only help camouflage areas where the leather's color has faded due to use and abuse.

CLEAN IT UP

Even if you never set your purse down on the floor of a restaurant, it can still get filthy. And since dropping your bag off at the purse dry cleaner is not a thing yet, you're going to have to clean it yourself.

Your first step in cleaning a leather bag that is only slightly dirty should be taking a baby wipe to it, making sure the wipes don't contain alcohol. Alcohol can damage leather, so use wipes meant for real baby bums, since they are much gentler. Take care not to soak the purse, since this can remove the protective coating on a real leather bag. If your bag is faux leather or plastic, feel free to go to town on it with any sort of wet wipe—it can take it.

One of the first bags I ever spent big money on was a light-colored, coated cotton canvas number from a fancy designer. After only one night of carrying it, I realized that my blue jeans had transferred dye all over my brand new bag, staining it terribly. I wish I could tell you my secret fix, but the sad truth is that there is actually no way to completely undo this disaster. I had a little luck using a makeup wipe (since it contains cleanser meant to gently remove gunk and grime), rubbing the area in a circular pattern, and then wiping with a dry cloth between applications, but it only did so much. I took another crack at it with a magic eraser (which is meant for cleaning kitchens and bathrooms, making it a bit abrasive—so I wouldn't try this on a leather bag), and it helped a little. But the end result is that the bag is still stained to this day, so your best bet is to take extra care when carrying a light-colored bag while wearing dark-colored clothing.

If your bag is made of suede, don't ever get it wet when attempting to clean it. Instead, brush off ground-in dirt with a suede brush, available at any shoe repair spot for about seven bucks. In a pinch, you can also use any brush with natural bristles—I once got a ton of ground-in birthday cake out of a klutzy actor's many-thousand-dollar suede clutch using the soft-bristled boars-hair brush I happen to always carry in my own personal handbag.

When cleaning your bag, don't overlook the metal hardware. It can easily get dull, dirty, and gunky from things like smoke, hand lotion, and hairspray residue. Give your bag's metal hardware a regular once-over with a double-sided jewelry cloth, and it will gleam as bright as the day you bought it. One side (usually the lighter-colored side) has a cleaning compound meant to take off any grease or grime—while the other side polishes and shines the newly clean surface. Jewelry cloths are available at any better jewelry store for about ten bucks, and a single one will last your entire life.

STORE IT

Is there any accessory more annoying to store than a bunch of purses? They vary too much in size and shape to really make any order of them, and existing storage systems for purchase at those organizing stores take up way too much space. But there are a few things you can do to make some sense of the mess.

TREAT 'EM RIGHT

Hanging bags by their handles can cause them to stretch and warp, so don't store them that way if you can help it. But ignore all those blogs that tell you to display your purses openly around the house as some sort of art—because dust and sunlight are the twin enemies of handbags, and exposure to them will significantly shorten the life of good and cheap purses alike. Those fancy dust bags come with expensive purses for a reason—and even less pricey bags will benefit from being stored away in a pouch that allows them to breathe while still being protected from the elements. If you don't own any purses that came with felt bags, don't worry: I just use old pillowcases to store bags that didn't come with their own protective covers. If you've got super-fancy bags you're looking to protect, your best bet is to stuff them with acid-free tissue paper (regular tissue paper gets acidic and brittle with age, and can transfer color onto adjacent objects) so they maintain their shape—then stash them away in non-airtight boxes (cardboard is best) so air can move freely through them, keeping them from drying out and rotting prematurely. If you live somewhere even a little bit humid, pop one of those silica packets (those things you get with most new shoes and bags that beseech you "DO NOT EAT!") in your fanciest bags—they'll last longer for it.

STUFF 'EM

Stuffing your purses when not in use will help them maintain their shape, keeping the sides from caving in on themselves and creating creases you can never get out. You can use acid-free tissue paper, but I like to just use a sweater or T-shirt I'm not currently wearing. (This is also a good use for worn-out clothes that aren't in good enough shape for a charity shop to sell.)

SORT BY OCCASION

Sort and separate purses according to the occasions you carry them: work, play, travel, and evening. I can't believe I didn't do this years ago—it's made my life so much easier! It has also encouraged me to finally get around to regularly using more of the bags I've obsessively collected over the years.

KEEP ODORS AT BAY

To keep your bags and purses smelling fresh, toss a dryer sheet inside each one before you stash it back on the shelf. It will keep musty smells from setting in when a purse is un-used for a long time, and it will also kill any smelly spill that may befall your favorite handbag. As an individual who is constantly putting iced lattes with wonky lids in her purse "for later," I can personally vouch for the dryer sheet's effectiveness.

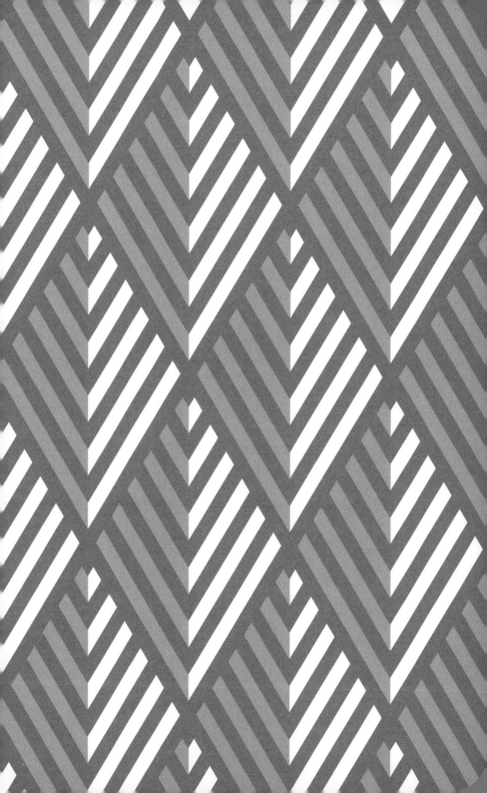

Yes, I'm Suggesting You Carry a Parasol

If you want to make it through the summer without looking like one of the California Raisins, you really should consider carrying a parasol to protect yourself from the scorching sun. I know it seems as if it would be hard to pull off without being costume-y, but as long as you are carrying your parasol outside in the sun (and not while strolling through an air-conditioned shopping mall), it is performing an actual function—and is therefore exempt from the normal rules of fashion and style. It's all about treating it as if it were just a fun afterthought—albeit one that just so happens to look adorable with what you casually threw on that day. I'll give you some parasol styling ideas below, but the only "rule" you need to follow when carrying one is to avoid clocking passersby with it—and to always be aware of the extra space a parasol takes up. They aren't really a great idea in a packed crowd or at a busy street fair, because you'll need plenty of room in order to properly twirl your parasol to your heart's content—without taking someone's eye out in the process.

PAPER IS BEST

I like a paper parasol for a myriad of reasons, but mainly because it's the most casual parasol available—and it doesn't call a lot of attention to itself. Plus, if you lose it, you're only out about eight bucks, so there's no real heartbreak. A loose, printed dress, classic straw tote, and a single piece of eye-catching jewelry is the best way to elevate a lowly paper parasol to star status.

GO FOR CROCHET

A sweet way to sport a Victorian-style, crocheted parasol in an off-white shade is to pair it with a simple round-necked T-shirt, floral printed shorts, a pair of wood-heeled sandals, and some dainty jewelry. If you're feeling a bit bolder, go for a goth-princess vibe by carrying a black crocheted parasol with a louche street-wear tee, denim pencil skirt, shiny sandals, and rocker-chic fringed bag.

POINTY PAGODA

Carrying a pointy, pagoda-shaped parasol (meant to mimic the ornamental structures found all over Asia in parks and gardens) is a lot of look. That's not to say you can't successfully pull it off, but just be aware that when your parasol is making a big, pointed statement, you want to make sure the rest of your outfit whispers. A plain T-shirt dress, cheeky tote bag, bow-bedecked flat sandals, and sparkly button earrings will do the trick nicely, allowing the parasol to be the high point of your ensemble.

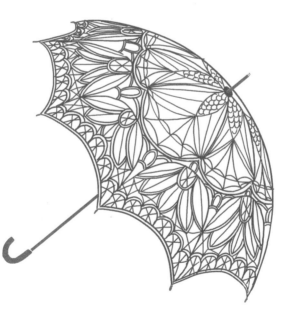

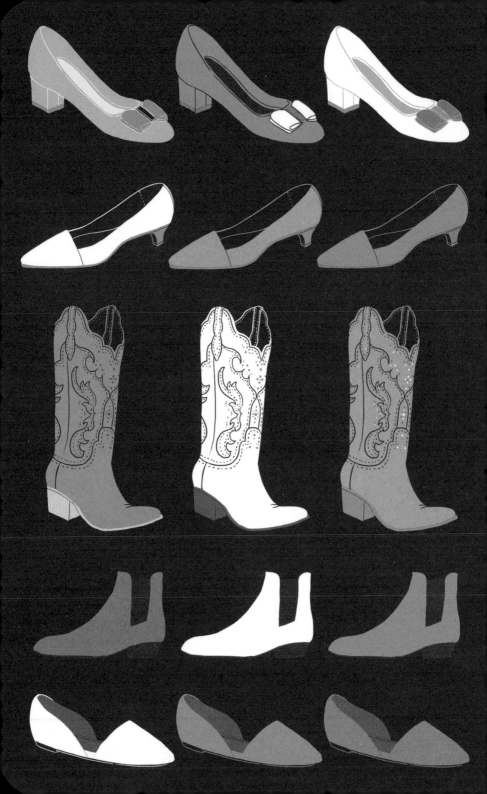

CHAPTER 6

SHOES

A Friend of the Foot

Shoes are the hardest-working, most practical accessories you own. Not only can you not live without them, they are functional devices that help you navigate through the world. Think about it: a necklace doesn't provide the foundation that holds your body up, a purse can't protect you from stubbing your toe, and a scarf won't ever help you chase down a taxicab. Not only do shoes work hard to protect your feet (and get you where you're going), they are also one of the easiest ways to change up (or completely ruin) an outfit lickety-split.

The old saying is that you can tell a lot about a person by their shoes, but I think that idea is actually kind of bunk—because it's always possible that the reason someone has muddy shoes is because they just pulled a drowning dog out of a lake. Besides, you can learn a lot more about someone by the way they treat waiters.

GET THE BALANCE RIGHT

Balance is the most important part of an ensemble, and shoes are the quickest way to either throw it off—or instantly correct it. To get

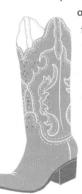

an idea of what I mean, take a good look at your outfit (head to toe) in a full-length mirror. Then, squint your eyes as you look at yourself—so you can only see basic shapes and colors. (It's a bit like narrowing the aperture on a camera, which is what photographers do to give themselves tight focus.) Once you've reduced your view to just those shapes and colors, ask yourself: Are those shapes and colors pleasing? A well-balanced outfit requires the right combination of many things—shape, form, pattern, height, style, color, texture, weight, and contrast—and your shoe choice is a big part of the balance equation.

After you've spent some time considering your outfit, ask yourself: What does it seem to need when you squint? If it's weight, add a pair of shoes with some heft—like a platform wedge. If it's shape (which will usually be obvious because your outfit will seem to have too many straight, square lines), go for a pair of shoes that have a bit of curve to them. If your outfit seems to be doing just fine on its own, what you may need is a pair of shoes that don't add any extra visual information to the mix—so you'd do well to slip on the least busy, most streamlined pair you own. A thin-soled ballet flat, or a sandal with razor-thin straps in a neutral color, will cause the eye to gloss right over them, making your clothes the focal point of your outfit (instead of your shoes). If your outfit seems to be lacking a little something that you can't quite pinpoint, what's missing may be contrast—so try a pair of shocking red cowboy boots or animal-print sandals. Your shoes will then become the star of your look, guaranteeing they will be the first thing people notice when you walk into a room.

This advice about balance is just to get you started—because there's really no blanket, cookie-cutter answer to which exact shoes to wear with an outfit. But with practice, you can train your eye to see just what sort of shoe an ensemble needs to get the balance right. It's not so much about having the "right" shoe, it's about how it all comes together on you as a whole that makes a shoe the correct shoe for your look—and for your personal style. Once you figure it out, you'll suddenly always know what pair of shoes looks—and works—best with whatever you happen to be wearing.

AN INCONVENIENT SHOE

Here's a fun fact about actors who wear high heels in movies or on TV shows: every single one of them secretly has a pair of Uggs, slippers, or flip-flops stashed somewhere near the set so they can take those painful heels off between takes. When I was a totally green costumer designer just starting out, my main job was to stand behind the camera, ready to pounce every time the director yelled "cut," because once they stopped rolling, I'd scurry forward with my actors' comfort shoes in my outstretched hands. They would descend upon me, tossing their heels aside and accepting their slippers with elaborate thanks and appreciation, as if I were presenting them with an Oscar. Stars really are just like us—because no matter what you do for a living, if your feet hurt, no part of your day is going to turn out right.

High heels have become shorthand for sexy, but they originally existed for a slightly gross, more practical purpose: Egyptian butchers wore them in order to walk over the bodies of the animals they were slaughtering so the blood didn't get on their feet. (If you keep that visual in mind the next time you are swooning over a pair of stilettos, they might not seem so alluring.) Your feet are the base of your body, so it should come as no surprise that high heels can affect your entire skeleton. A little high-heel wearing is okay, but they just aren't designed for all-day wear, no matter what a bunch of fashion mags may try to tell you. Even if you don't feel pain when you wear them, high heels are actively ruining your feet. They shift your weight to the balls of your feet—causing your knees and hips to tilt forward. At the same time, you're forced to lean backward in order to maintain your balance (the wobbly imbalance of wearing heels is actually the reason your butt looks so good in them, by the way), and this all eventually leads to extra stress on your knees, joints, hips, and back—not to mention the dangers of developing bunions, ingrown toenails, and calluses due to your feet being constantly pushed forward. And what if you suddenly need to run, jump, kick, or fight? It's hard to do that in heels unless you are an action-movie heroine.

THINK YOU HAVE TO WEAR HEELS AT WORK? THINK AGAIN

You may think that in order to be office-appropriate and meet your business's dress code, you must wear heels. But the current guidelines of the United States Equal Employment Opportunity Commission (the federal agency that administers and enforces laws against workplace discrimination) are pretty clear: dress code restrictions must be pertinent to a job and can't require more of one gender than the other. That means all you need to be appropriate in a formal work setting is footwear that has a certain amount of polish and a high level of smartness, no matter the heel height. It sounds good on paper, but the options available to women for formal dress shoes that aren't heels are shockingly minimal—and you really have to dig, scrounge, and search in order to find them.

ALTERNATIVES TO HIGH HEELS

The key to making a pair of flats or low-heeled shoes right for any fancy occasion (or on the job) is to pay attention to the level of refinement. That means if you're looking for shoes to wear with a work ensemble, it's best to seek out styles in patent leather or smooth, highly polished, flat leather, since suede and fabric can tend to look more casual. If you're headed to a fancy party, pairs that have some embellishment, sheen, or sparkle will instantly make them appear more formal. Keep in mind that a shoe with a thinner ankle strap will also naturally add a sense of fanciness, helping to make your overall look way dressier. Avoid thick rubber-soled shoes, as they will likely lack the level of formality you're looking for. If you want to sidestep the problem of wearing heels to a fancy event altogether, just wear a really long dress—because if nobody can see your feet, it's quite easy to wear a flat shoe without it being too obvious.

The first few times you wear flat shoes when you'd normally wear heels, it may feel as if you're not exactly pulling it off, but the truth is that they probably look way cuter than you think—it just takes a while for your eye to get used to seeing something new. If you're searching for shoes to replace heels, try one of the options below. Your hooves will thank you for it.

D'ORSAY FLATS: These are shoes in which the inside portion (usually on both sides) of the shoe has been cut away, revealing the arch of the foot. Named after the Count d'Orsay (a French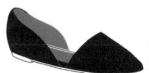

gadabout and fashion dandy) in the 1800s, d'Orsay flats have that all-important extra bit of interest that makes them a perfect replacement for high heels in a conservative workplace that requires closed-toe shoes.

BLOCK HEELS: Shoe wizard Roger Vivier turned the footwear world on its head in 1965 with his playful, modern take on the pilgrim shoe—a low block-heeled number called the Belle Vivier. Famously worn by Catherine Deneuve in the film *Belle de Jour*, the block-heeled shoe trend dovetailed perfectly with the mid-1960s women's rights movement. Since they're easy to walk in, far more stable than a pair of stilettos, and don't get stuck in subway grates, block heels have not gone out of style since.

KITTEN HEELS: Yes, the lowly kitten heel has been much maligned over the years, but the truth is they are actually a godsend, since sometimes even the tiniest heel can help a pair of pants look as if they're the proper length, saving you from spending a ton of money on tailoring. But the really great thing about kitten heels (besides the fact that your feet will thank you) is that because they are naturally a more subdued, conservative shoe, you have license to go a little wild with the rest of your outfit.

MENSWEAR-STYLE OXFORDS: These have been in and out of style since the mid-1970s, and some folks seem to think they can't wear oxfords and still look cute due to their somewhat masculine style. But the trick to making them work is to either embrace the masculinity—styling them with very androgynous pieces—or balancing out that masculinity with something ultra-feminine, like a ruffled blouse. If you think you can't wear oxfords because they make your legs look stumpy, try styling them with tights or stockings. It effectively hides where they cut you off at the ankle, creating a nice, clean, unbroken line. And if you think oxfords can't work for evenings, think again: when paired with sheer colored stockings or fishnets, they are as alluring as any pair of high heels. Printed oxfords (such as cheetah or plaid) can seem hard to style, but the rules of pattern mixing for clothes hold true with shoes, too: just pair them with a pattern in both the same color family and of the same size or scale, and you'll be golden.

SMOKING SLIPPERS: My very favorite shoes are a pair of black velvet smoking slippers with gold scorpions embroidered on the toes that I stole from a teenage boy. He was playing Othello on a show I was the costume designer for, and we happened to wear the same shoe size—so when the show had a wardrobe sale at the end of the season, I snapped them up, not realizing at the time that they were the high heel alternative I'd been searching for my entire life.

Smoking slippers originally functioned solely as an upper-crust house shoe (an indoor replacement for outdoor footwear) because roads in Victorian England were made of gravel and sand that tended to mar the expensive rugs and flooring of the landed gentry's homes. In modern times, velvet smoking slippers are the perfect replacement for high heels, since they add a rich sense of fancy entitlement to any outfit you pair them with. And if you have a larger foot and can wear shoes available only in men's sizes (usually a women's size eight and up), you're in luck—because some of the fanciest, cleverest smoking slippers the world has to offer are made exclusively for men.

BACKLESS LOAFER MULE: Gucci mastermind Alessandro Michele's greatest gift to the world is his clever resurrection of a 1990s classic: the backless loafer/mule hybrid. It's the mullet of shoes: business in the front and party in the back. The inherent classicism of a loafer-style shoe adds instant polish to anything you pair them with (and easily answers the question of what to wear to work when you can't show your toes), but you also can slide them off under your desk anytime you like—and nobody will be the wiser.

SNEAKERS: The trend of wearing sneakers with a work or nighttime look may seem kind of haphazard, but peek a little closer and you'll start to notice that those fashionable peeps who seem to oh-so-casually match a pair of sneakers with a fancier ensemble have actually given their look a lot of extra thought. They haven't chosen just any sneaker—they've selected their kicks as they would any other footwear: to echo or reinforce specific elements of their outfit, such as color, 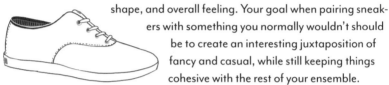 shape, and overall feeling. Your goal when pairing sneakers with something you normally wouldn't should be to create an interesting juxtaposition of fancy and casual, while still keeping things cohesive with the rest of your ensemble.

To make sneakers work with a dress or fancy slacks, look for pairs that are a bit more refined. A light dusting of sparkle and gems will instantly up the fancy factor, as will a pair with soles that are the same color as the uppers, since a lot of what makes a sneaker fancy-dress-worthy is simply the thickness of the sole. There's an exception to every rule, of course, but an easy guideline is that the thinner the sole, the more refined the sneaker likely looks. And remember: as with any new fashion thing you try, it always takes a minute for your eyes to get used to seeing it.

SHOW SOME SKIN FOR LONGER LEGS

Successfully wearing flat shoes with outfits that traditionally call for a heel involves creating flattering proportions—since showing the right amount of skin will automatically lengthen and enhance your silhouette. Pairing low-contrast sandals (white or pastels for pale skin tones, black or burgundy for darker) with a shorter garment is an easy way to get comfortable with wearing flats, since the combination immediately makes your legs look longer. Showing a bit more skin offsets the stumpy feeling flats can sometimes give you—and whether you realize it or not, leg lengthening is what your eye mainly reacts to when you slip on high heels and decide you like the look. Exposing your kneecaps is more than enough skin for this formula to work, so there's no need to force yourself into a miniskirt situation if that's not your bag.

Low-heeled or flat shoes work well with either very short or all-the-way-to-the-floor dresses and skirts, but pieces that hit you at midknee or midcalf can be challenging, as they don't show quite enough skin—and can tend to cut off the leg line abruptly. A good way to combat this is to wear garments that have side vents, which give the illusion of a shorter hemline when you walk, since the vent opens up and exposes more skin. Asymmetrical hemlines are another good choice, as the jagged, uneven hemline helps add to the illusion by confusing the eye as to where the leg actually begins and ends.

CONSIDER YOUR VAMP

You can also create the appearance of a longer leg by wearing a shoe with a low vamp, also known as the part of the shoe that covers your toes. A low vamp ends just above your toes (or even offers some toe cleavage, which is truly the grossest turn of phrase ever)—while a high vamp extends to cover the area close to your ankle. Low-vamped shoes that show a lot of foot are ideal with skirts, dresses, and cropped pants—all of which are famous for chopping up the leg visually, making it appear stumpy or short. Classic low-vamped shoes include thongs, ballet flats, and pumps, but knee-high boots actually perform close to the same function, since they create a long, unbroken line on the leg from your toes all the way up to your knees.

CAN I SHOW MY TOES AT WORK?

It really depends on your workplace, but an easy way to never be too casual at work is to never show your toes on the job—so it's a good idea to have at least one pair of sandals that covers your toes completely in your office-duty shoe wardrobe.

MIX AND MATCH

Contrasting your shoes with your outfits is highly encouraged these days, since getting all matchy-matchy is almost totally a thing of the past, but it's easy to get overwhelmed by the possibility of overdoing it—so it's a good idea to have some tricks up your sleeve until it becomes second nature.

MATCH A LITTLE SOMETHING, ANYTHING

Match your shoes with your earrings, a bracelet, or even the tiniest bit of color in a pattern on your skirt. It doesn't matter how small it is, since the simple act of repeating a color will help your shoe choice make instant sense.

MATCH WITH TEXTURE

Try a pair of shoes that has the same amount of texture as something else in your outfit, like a pair of fishnet tights matched with snakeskin ankle boots or a nubby tweed skirt. The two patterns work together nicely because they are obviously different—yet still reminiscent of each other.

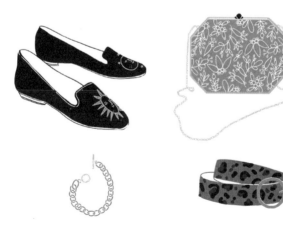

TRAVELING WITH SHOES: THE WORST!

I am always thrilled to go on vacation until I have to start packing my shoes—then it hits me like a ton of bricks that there is no way in hell I can fit everything I want to bring in my suitcase unless I seriously edit down my shoe choices. The best solution to this problem is to decide before you leave town what your main accessory color story will be for the trip (for me, it's always black or brown), which means you won't be tempted to pack a single thing that doesn't go with your black or brown belt, shoes, and purse. It helpfully forces you to pick clothes to go with your shoes—not the other way around. If you are traveling for a wedding or other special event, you obviously may have to take an extra pair that goes with your special attire, but otherwise, packing around a single shoe and accessory color story lightens your load instantly.

THE THREE-SHOE WEEKEND

I'm sure there are those who can manage to take a weekend trip and only bring one single pair of shoes, but I'm never going to be that person. However, three pairs of shoes are likely the max you should allow yourself to bring (flip-flops for the pool and slippers for warmth notwithstanding)—and since you'll be wearing one pair on the journey there, you'll really only need to pack two of them. Here's a blueprint for the ideal three-shoe wardrobe, suitable for any weekend jaunt:

ONE WORKHORSE SHOE FOR HEAVY WALKING: If you're not sure what works best for this purpose, start experimenting—because the time to figure out what shoes you can walk ten-plus miles or more in is not in the middle of a trip. My workhorse walkers are a pair of Blundstone ankle boots with red contrast soles. They look just as good with rolled up jeans as they do with tights and dresses, and if I wind up having to wear them out to dinner, I compensate with heaps of sparkly rhinestone jewelry to bump up the fancy factor. I'm always the envy of my fellow travelers when I can still walk fifteen blocks at the end of a long day without hobbling.

ONE SHOE THAT IS A LITTLE NICER (BUT STILL COMFY): This might be a low wedge that could go out to dinner—and also take a light midnight walking tour of the area's attractions. You won't need to walk ten miles in these shoes, but they shouldn't be a pair of painful car-to-restaurant shoes only—since shoes you can't trek in have no place on vacation. Absolutely nobody looks cute holding their heels in their hands as they walk down the street at 1:00 a.m.

ONE WILD CARD: This is your place to go crazy. Will they be the special heels for the event that is the reason for the weekend in the first place? Or are they workout sneakers because you are a person who likes to hit the hotel gym? Maybe they are a pair of jeweled slides that go *so well* with that one dress you want to wear to dinner that you'll allow yourself the luxury of packing them for one-time use only? It's totally up to you.

HOW TO PACK 'EM

Always, always pack your shoes away in something: be it a shoe bag, felt bag from a handbag purchase, old pillowcase, mesh bag, or lowly plastic grocery bag. When I'm packing my actors' suitcases for location shoots and press junkets where they'll be taking care of their wardrobe on their own, I pack each individual shoe in its own bag so I can sneakily cram them into every available nook and cranny in their suitcases, since a full pair in a bag together takes up way too much room. Putting shoes in a bag for travel also conveniently covers dirty soles, which helps keep your clothes from getting filthy when they wind up crammed next to them.

FLIP-FLOPS: YAY OR NAY?

Among the most boring and hotly debated topics on the Internet is when (or where) flip-flops are acceptable footwear. The answer depends on where you're headed to. But I'm not sure what other style of shoe you'd wear to the beach or swimming pool, and when you're not at work (unless you're a lifeguard). There's absolutely no reason you can't wear flip-flops during your daily routine. A trip to the grocery store, gas station, post office, coffee shop, or dry cleaner all count as flip-flop-friendly scenarios. But none of this is to say that you can't also successfully wear a pair of rubber flip-flops to a bar with a vintage 1950s prom dress and totally rule the roost style-wise—because I sure have. In your off-duty life, anything that makes you feel cool and good about yourself is a go. But there are a few places where flip-flops probably aren't such a great idea.

PLACES YOU MOST DEFINITELY SHOULD NOT WEAR FLIP-FLOPS:

» Any restaurant with cloth napkins

» Religious services (unless they're in a revival tent)

» Red carpet events

» Funerals (yes, even if they're held outdoors)

» First date or blind date (unless it's at the beach; then have at it)

» Business meetings

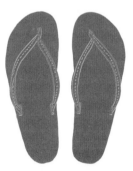

OLD SHOE JAZZ

If you're bored with your current shoes but don't have the money to replace them all and start again (and who among us does?), try one of these tricks to jazz them up for almost zero dollars instead.

SPRAY PAINT 'EM

In a fit of desperation on a commercial shoot, I once spray painted an actor's heels to match her outfit. Thinking the shoes would only last for the one shoot day, I let her take them home—only to be shocked when I ran into her a year later at a party, where she was still wearing those same heels I'd sprayed with dollar-store paint. This story illustrates that clearly, any old can of spray paint will do, but you'd probably get even longer-lasting wear if you use spray paint specifically meant for leather, vinyl, or plastic (such as Nu-Life, Brillo, or Magix color spray). No matter what type of paint you use, here are a few tips to keep in mind for a better outcome:

» Spray paint will adhere quite well if you dull down the surface of the shoes before painting. Apply a bit of nail polish remover (the kind containing acetone) to the exterior of the shoe with a cotton ball, rubbing briskly until the shine disappears or the shoe takes on a dull appearance.

» Spray lightly with long, even, sweeping motions, and keep in mind that three thin coats will wear better than one or two thicker coats. Allow each coat to dry for one hour between applications.

» To create a smooth painting surface (which will help cut down on streaks and drips), stuff the toes of the shoes you are painting with newspaper or plastic bags so they retain their shape.

» If you are using a metallic color, first apply a nonmetallic base coat in a similar or lighter color to act as a primer; this will provide more complete color coverage, since some metallic paints tend to go on thinly.

LOOK TO LACES

The fastest way to give a beefed-up pair of shoes new life is to swap your laces out for either a fresh, new, unfrayed pair—or for a colorful, fanciful pair that will totally switch up their original style. Laces are measured in inches, so knowing the length of your original laces is the easiest way to make sure your new pair will fit.

ATTEMPT SOME ART

Can you draw? Can your BFF? If so, decorating an inexpensive pair of plain white canvas sneakers with your favorite sports team's logo, a portrait of your dog, or an inside joke is a fun way to make something that is memorable, personal, unique, and best of all: inexpensive. Acrylic paint works best on canvas, and things will look even better if you take the time to prepare the shoes with an acrylic-based primer beforehand.

EARRINGS AREN'T JUST FOR EARS

If you've ever seen a unique pair of vintage earrings in a store and bemoaned the fact that they were the old-school clip-on type, don't fret—because you can put them to far better use by pressing them into service as a pair of shoe clips. When clipped onto the vamp of a pair of pumps, across the laces of a sneaker, or onto a thin, delicate sandal strap, clip-on earrings are a cute way to make any plain pair of shoes seem a little more special.

WHAT MAKES A CHEAP SHOE GREAT?

Sometimes, even the richest babe in the world will need to wear an inexpensive pair of shoes—because no matter how much money you have, if you just want to partake in a shoe trend that you know you won't care about six months from now, a cheaper version will usually do. This is especially true if you need a pair of pumps just for one-time wear, but don't want to look as if you purchased them at the dollar store.

If so, follow these tips for faking a lesser shoe into one that looks like it cost way more—and nobody will ever be the wiser:

» Choose a shoe in either fabric or faux suede instead of fake leather. Smooth, artificial leather almost always looks unrealistic, but intricate brocade boots, suede-look ballet flats, or satin-esque slides somehow manage to look a bit fancier.

» Another good cheat is to pick a pair with a heel that matches the upper part of the shoe. Those stacked wooden heels are fine on a brown shoe—but on a black or brightly colored pair, they draw needless attention to the feet, causing a cheaper pair of shoes to be examined more closely than you might like.

» Any pair of shoes that has some sort of decorative stitching, contrasting piping, elaborate embroidery, or other embellishments usually looks far fancier than they really are—since those are the classical hallmarks of more expensive shoes.

WHY THE MOST EXPENSIVE SHOES SOMETIMES STINK

Soon after getting my very first costume design job, I sprang for a pair of red velvet Prada platform sandals I'd seen touted in an issue of *Vogue* as the season's must-have. I scrimped and saved and finally took my money—in the form of crumpled $20 bills in a Mason jar (I was so green, I didn't even have a credit card!)—to the Prada store in Beverly Hills and bought the shoes, cost be damned. Not only did those shoes instantly cut my feet to ribbons, every single strap on them soon broke in rapid succession. I dutifully took them to my shoe repair guy, who carefully hammered each strap back in place with tiny little nails. A few months later, I opened up the September issue of *Vogue* only to find those same red velvet Prada sandals now on their "Out" list for fall. I instantly felt foolish but didn't realize just how badly I'd been played until years later. Spending more money on something doesn't always guarantee quality—and sometimes, what you are paying for is simply an illusion. So before you spend a bundle on a pair of shoes, make sure you know how to spot a truly well-made pair.

LOOK FOR FULL-GRAIN LEATHER: Full-grain leather is made from a hide that has been only minimally treated. It has not endured harsh chemical treatments and so with care, should age well and last for years. You should be able to clearly see the grain and pores of the leather on a pair of full-grain leather shoes.

Most shoes are made of corrected leather, which has been sanded down to remove imperfections and then coated with sealant. You won't be able to see the tiny pores of the hide when you look closely, since they've been sanded away and dulled over with the sealant. With wear, corrected leather shoes will eventually crease and peel. Most shoes you own will be made of corrected leather, and that's fine! Just don't get suckered into paying huge bucks for them.

CHECK THE SOLES: The soles of a costly pair of shoes should be bonded securely. A really well made shoe will have a sole that is stitched into place—as well as being glued. If a shoe sports a sole affixed only with adhesive, it will eventually come unglued and start flapping as you walk. And if you notice globs of glue oozing out from where the sole meets the upper part of the shoe, they aren't worth the money. Not only is it unsightly, excess glue eventually causes the shoe to separate and fall apart—and there isn't any good fix for it.

STICK YOUR HANDS INSIDE: Make sure the insole of a shoe you are considering purchasing isn't wrinkled or bubbling up anywhere. A bad insole is a telltale sign of a poor-quality shoe. Look out for rough-edges or stick-on labels inside the shoe, since very well made shoes will have their labels stitched to the insole.

DOES IT PASS THE SMELL TEST?: If costly shoes happen to smell like burning tires, they aren't worth the cash. Really good shoes have a pleasing scent that calls to mind leather, polish, and wood.

LISTEN CLOSELY: Try walking in any shoes you plan to buy on a hard surface before you commit—not just on the plush carpet of most shoe departments. Squeaky sounds are a dead giveaway of subpar shoes. Also, keep an ear out for wedges and platforms that sound hollow inside.

FORGET A CRUMMY ZIPPER: Zippers that don't zip up smoothly and easily will eventually break—and replacing a zipper on a shoe is an annoying, costly proposition.

CHECK THE HEEL CAPS: Stiletto caps that aren't tightly secured to the heel will soon come loose, exposing the heel spike—which can result not only in it being ground down as you walk (a condition that isn't easily repairable), but can also make it dangerous to traipse on smooth surfaces without slipping and falling. (If you find yourself with a lost stiletto heel cap in a pinch, you can temporarily cover the exposed spike with a pen cap. Just choose one that has a flat top, not a pointy one.)

BEWARE OF BITS AND BOBS THAT ARE READY TO FALL OFF: Embellishments (such as rhinestones) that aren't properly secured are a sure sign that not enough care went into the making of a pair of shoes, and getting a heavy-duty needle and thread into the cramped space inside of a shoe to fasten them is tedious at best— and impossible at worst.

ONLINE HUNTING: EFFECTIVE VINTAGE SHOE SEARCH TERMS

Vintage shoes can present a pickle—you'll usually find a million great styles, but since shoes are regularly subjected to rain, snow, pavement pounding, and foot sweat, they tend to take a severe beating along the way. I'm wary of buying any vintage shoes that predate the 1970s, since they are usually at the end of their useful lives. Straps and buckles are the first things that break—and leather tends to dry out and crack, rendering the entire shoe useless. Proceed with caution when considering the purchase of vintage shoes. Although there are a few repairs you can easily do, for the most part, it's buyer beware. Here are a few brands that tend to hold up well over time, so are worth seeking out online:

FERRAGAMO: The classic rich-lady shoe is a pair of low-heeled pumps with a flat grosgrain bow at the toe, topped off with a flat metal disk stamped Ferragamo. Called the Vara, these shoes have been in style ever since their introduction in 1978, and they still retail for four to five hundred dollars brand new. They are almost indestructible, so if you find a vintage pair in your size, snap them up post-haste! Style your Varas with colored or printed tights for a dash of funky—yet ladylike—pizzazz.

FRYE BOOTS: Originally designed in 1863 for factory workers in New England, Frye boots managed to become uber-stylish somewhere along the way—and have since been worn by everyone from Jackie O. to Bruce Springsteen. In the 1960s, Frye introduced the Campus boot (a fourteen- to fifteen-inch-tall boot with a bulky toe and chunky heel), and it is no stretch to say that the Campus was the ultimate fashion boot throughout the 1960s and 1970s. It came in a variety of colors, but banana (a pale yellowy-tan shade) was the most popular. Finding a vintage pair of Frye boots is a score—because even if the soles are shot, once they are replaced, the boots are as good as new. When it comes to replacement soles for Frye boots, Vibram soles are the gold standard—so accept no substitutes.

WORISHOFER: If you've ever had a hankering for grandma-style sandals, you probably had a pair of Worishofers in mind. Born in Germany, these sensible-cute sandals have existed as shock-absorbing marvels since the 1940s, but they've recently reemerged as part of the style ethos that champions ugly as the new adorable. Modern versions mirror vintage ones almost exactly, so grab an older pair in any color you can manage to find. They liven up a T-shirt and jeans more than a pair of sneakers ever could—and are even nice enough to wear with a church-going sundress.

FAMOLARE: This company reinvented footwear in the late 1970s with the Get There shoe, a clog style that turned the platform shoe trend on its head by using a newfangled wave sole. It promoted good posture and proper balance by shifting your body weight across the entire foot instead of forcing it forward onto the toes—resulting in platform shoes you could actually walk in. Famolare disappeared from the market sometime in the late 1980s or early 1990s, but relaunched in 2017 with price points around one hundred and fifty dollars—making well-kept vintage versions more than worth the money.

COLLECTIBLE COWBOY BOOTS: Vintage cowboy boots are better than modern versions in almost every way. They are usually better made—and way more stylish. Brands to keep an eye out for include Lucchese, Nocona, Acme, Dingo, Dan Post, Tony Lama, and Justin.

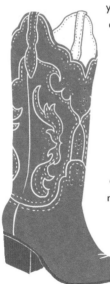

Just be careful to ensure the pair you've got your eye on isn't made with exotic skins from an endangered species. While vintage boots are obviously secondhand and your purchase doesn't directly support poaching, buying them may still be illegal. If you wind up with a pair of cowboy boots that are a bit too big or small, try them on with a different pair of socks before giving up. Thick wool socks will make a pair of too-big boots seem a half-size smaller, while a pair of tights or stockings will help your foot and ankle slide in and out of a too-small pair far more easily.

THREE EASY FIXES FOR VINTAGE SHOES

Buying a pair of vintage shoes practically guarantees you'll be forced to fix at least a little something somewhere along the way. Lots of problems with older shoes render them beyond repair, but if a pair you've got your eye on only needs one of the simple fixes below, you're golden.

STOP A FLAPPING BOTTOM

If the sole of a vintage shoe is flapping or loose, it can likely be put back in place with a bit of Shoe Goo, an adhesive meant specifically for shoes that allows for flexibility (unlike regular glue, which is rigid once dry). But heed some advice that I'm always too impatient to follow: let the glue cure for a full twenty-four hours before attempting to walk out the door.

REPLACE THE INSIDE

If the inside of a vintage shoe is discolored and gross, you can cover it easily with a thin pair of insoles from the drugstore. If there isn't enough space left over for your foot once you pop in a new insole, consider removing the existing ruined insole so you can replace it with your store-bought one.

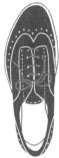

REINCARNATE OLD SOLES

If the bottoms of a pair of vintage shoes are worn down, you may be able to successfully have a shoe repair shop resole them—but keep in mind that once a pair of shoes gets that far gone, they are likely at the end of their useful life anyway. You'd probably be fixing one thing only to have another (like a buckle or strap) break soon thereafter. But if all you're looking at is a slightly worn down heel or toe (as a result of someone who drags their feet when they walk), resoling is absolutely the best way to give an old pair of shoes a little more life—so go for it.

STORE IT

Save yourself a lot of time and take it from me: there is no absolutely perfect way to store shoes. They take up an annoying amount of space—and like anything that comes in a pair, keeping them together is a challenge. The fancy Hollywood actors that I've helped to organize their closets over the years love to have me store their shoes in the boxes they came in, with actual photos of the shoes taped to the outside. But in real life, nobody has time for that foolishness. I store my personal shoes in a multitude of ways, depending on their size and the frequency with which I wear them. The shoes I wear most live in an over-the-door shoe rack that I cover up with a curtain to protect them from dust, while my boots are stored in slide-front drawers underneath my hanging clothes. My sandals and ballet flats are neatly stashed in one of those space-saving, as-seen-on-TV underbed shoe storage things that I can easily pull out anytime I need.

If you have zero space or cash to dedicate to official shoe storage, squeezing a thrift-store bookshelf into a corner and stashing your shoes in pairs (alternating heel to toe to save valuable inches) is your best bet; just tack a curtain panel or piece of cute fabric to the front so they don't get dusty from exposure to the elements. The fabric can then be easily tied back with a piece of ribbon when you are perusing your collection and deciding what to wear.

The Big Three: Socks, Pantyhose, and Tights

Upgrading your foot coverings will make your boring old shoes suddenly feel brand new again—but if you're not used to viewing something as basic as a pair of socks, stockings, or tights as a fashion accessory, it can be hard to know where to start.

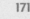

THE BEGINNER'S GUIDE TO SOCKING

Not enough of you fools are wearing socks. I know, because I've been forced to smell a million stinky, sockless, actors' feet over the years—and stars really are just like the rest of us: sometimes super-glam, sometimes kind of gross. Socks exist mainly to protect your feet from being rubbed raw by shoes and to act as extra insulation to keep your feet warm, but the real reason socks are important is that they keep your sweaty feet from stinking up and ruining your shoes. Socks also easily allow you to express personality even when your work-place has a staid, boring dress code—because who could complain about a sliver of a colorful sock showing when you cross your legs in a meeting and your pants creep up a bit at the ankle?

If you're not used to wearing socks for fashion only, ease your way into it by pairing interesting, meant-to-be-seen ones with your casual sneakers (or any shoe that has a sporty vibe to it). This look works because sporty shoes have an innately practical feeling to them—and apart from shoes, socks are the most practical accessories there are. This all means that you can feel free to wear socks that have a really whimsical vibe—and things will still look pretty basic and normal. Thinner, patterned ankle socks pair well with loafers for work, since the inherent sensibility of both also makes for a natural marriage.

As you experiment, if it feels as if a certain sock and shoe combo is starting to look a bit more whimsical than you imagined, don't fight it—embrace it! You'll eventually find the level of whimsy that works for you. Sometimes, sheer black socks with your work flats are as far as you can go, and that's fine. You are still adding a little bit of *je ne sais quoi* to your look with very little cost or effort and making your feet comfier to boot. Keeping your socks close to or directly in the same color family as your shoes is the safest route, but if you're feeling frisky, branch out and try some of the more daring styling equations below. (And remember: When socking strictly for fashion purposes, you'll want the lightest, thinnest, wispiest socks you can find. This is especially true if the shoe you're wearing is heavier—or covers a large portion of your foot.)

WHY DON'T YOU TRY . . .

» Cuffed jeans + canvas sneakers + animal-print socks

» Midi-length skirt + low block heels + fishnet socks

» Summer sundress + open-toe platforms + floral-patterned socks

» Menswear-style suit + brown loafers + trouser-length copper metallic socks

» Black cropped pants + white sandals + olive green socks

» Black-and-white outfit + gray- and white-patterned heels + red- and pink-patterned socks

» Party dress + cute strappy sandals + short rhinestone-embellished socks

KEEP YOUR SOCKS
FROM SLIP SLIDING AWAY

Wearing socks with heels sounds crazy cute until you try to walk somewhere and realize that heels have a natural tendency to push your foot forward, a condition that is exacerbated by adding slippery socks to the mix. Avoid socks that have slick bottoms if you're attempting to wear them with heels—or look for a set of thin, self-adhesive silicone or suede ball-of-foot halter inserts that will help keep your foot in place.

SOCKS AND ANKLE BOOTS: NATURAL-BORN ENEMIES

Wearing socks with ankle boots is annoying. No-show socks fall down mercilessly—and regular athletic socks can look dorky peeking out from sleek booties. Luckily, the solution to this vexing problem is easy: just wear socks that are 100 percent meant to be seen. Try a pair with some sort of cute detail at the ankle, such as lace, bows, polka dots, or even pointy kitty-cat ears.

If you loathe the idea of drawing even more attention to your ankles, strive to match your socks very closely to your boot color so they don't distract from the rest of your look. If all else fails, default to simple black ankle socks scrunched down inside your booties—they will easily blend into the dark, shadowy recess and make themselves almost invisible.

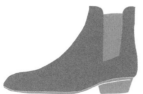
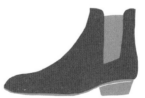

NOBODY WEARS PANTYHOSE ANYMORE, RIGHT?

The sheer leg coverings that we now call pantyhose first made an appearance in the 1920s, when they were called stockings. They were made of silk or rayon until late 1939, when nylon came on the scene. But World War II put the kibosh on nylon stocking production almost as soon as it had gotten started, because nylon factories had to switch to manufacturing materials for the war effort. Fashionable women of the 1940s temporarily had to make do instead with "Victory Hose," also known as leg makeup.

Covering your legs was part of every office dress code well into the late 1980s—but in the early 1990s, women started to rock bare legs with impunity. Now, we have an entire generation of women who are entering the workforce to whom it would never occur to purchase or wear a pair of flesh-toned pantyhose, ever—but if you hate shaving, dislike something about your legs, or are always a bit cold in the office, they can be a godsend. Pantyhose have improved dramatically in recent years and now come in versions that are light as air—yet still able to provide enough leg coverage to be worth the effort. If the look of bare legs isn't your jam (but you still want a bit of support), a pair of sheer black hose is the answer to all your problems. They make any skirt or dress seem instantly more office-appropriate (no matter how short it is) and are perfect to wear under pants to make undergarment lines disappear.

Wearing hose is also a good way to keep things neatly squared away with a slinky blouse and skirt—because if you tuck your top into the waistband of your hosiery, you won't find yourself retucking it in all day long. Tucking your blouse into your stockings is also pretty much the only way to stop those pesky shirt lines that run across your backside from being visible through your pants or skirt.

But don't misunderstand me: pantyhose are not de rigueur in any but the most conservative of professions—so unless you're a lawyer trying a landmark case against the tobacco industry, you needn't bother messing with them unless you want to. If I were to attend a dinner at Buckingham Palace where I was meant to meet the Queen of England, I'd probably wear a pair of sheer stockings just to feel completely dressed—but until that invite comes, I'll be bare-legging it at parties, weddings, and balls all across the land.

HOW TO MASTER WEARING TIGHTS

When the weather turns cold, even the bravest among us eventually has to submit to wearing tights to keep warm. Magazine editors and fancy New York types are photographed barelegged in January quite frequently, but their posh lives allow them to flit from lush townhouse to chauffeur-driven car to high-rise office building and back, never to find themselves standing on a street corner or subway platform with chattering teeth while waiting for a ride. If you live somewhere really, really, cold, look into getting yourself a pair of fleece-lined tights—they are like pants in stocking form and will keep you toasty warm, even in freezing rain or snow.

Wearing tights is a bit more challenging than regular hosiery, since they are a solid, opaque block of color that can tend to break up the natural flow of an outfit. I pretty much wear only black tights for this exact reason, but it is actually possible to wear interesting tights without looking like a toddler. The trick is to make sure you balance out the innate high-contrast look tights give an outfit by getting smart about what clothes you pair them with.

Try out some of these simple tights pairings for starters, and you'll soon understand what I mean:

BLACK-AND-WHITE HOUNDSTOOTH JACKET + RED OR BURGUNDY TIGHTS: Anything in the red family is a natural match for a black-and-white ensemble. It works because while black and white are neutrals on their own, adding a power color like red to the mix makes for an arresting look that is still a bit classic and conservative. It's an easy way to try something bold if you work in a staid office environment, since red always grabs a fair amount of attention—but houndstooth is a forever classic.

BLACK DRESS + STRIPED TIGHTS: Tights with stripes or other repeating patterns can be a lot for the eye to take in, so they are best paired with something simple like a plain black dress. But since striped tights pull so much focus, they are also a great way to wear that same black dress way more than once a week without anybody being the wiser.

CAMEL HAIR COAT + MUSTARD-HUED TIGHTS: This combo works because camel and mustard are in the same color family (which makes for a nice monochromatic pairing), yet are far enough apart on the spectrum (with camel leaning toward brown and mustard leaning toward yellow) to keep it from being too boring.

BRIGHT SHIFT DRESS + NEUTRAL GRAY TIGHTS: Sometimes a crazily colorful outfit needs a dose of slightly somber gray to tone things down a bit. But if the overall look starts to get a little too drab once you add in gray, try repeating one of the bright colors found in your dress with your shoes.

GRAY DRESSY SHORTS + BLACK PLAID TIGHTS: Wearing dressy shorts as an alternative to miniskirts is about the greatest going-out hack there is, but pairing them with solid black tights can tend to look too boring and serious. Instead, try a pair of plaid tights that perfectly play off of the casual vibe a pair of shorts naturally has.

STORE IT

Rolling your socks up into balls is likely how you've been storing them your entire life, but this method takes up far too much space—and will result in the elastic being stressed, which causes it to give out and become saggy in no time flat. Instead, fold your paired-up socks in half at the heel and lay them flat in your drawer. If you are a person who loses a sock to the wash every single time you do laundry without fail, do what I do with my actors' laundry on shows and safety pin your socks together before tossing them in the wash. You'll never wind up with a forlorn pile of lonely, single socks ever again.

Socks are easy enough to store neatly, but tights and pantyhose are a special kind of hell to keep organized. The Internet has a bunch of neurotic, time-consuming ways to store them, including stockpiling toilet paper rolls from the bathroom to tuck them neatly into, but I'm not all that interested in having anything that's been next to a toilet living in my lingerie drawer. After years of real-world testing, I can safely say that there are only a few ways to keep tights and panty-hose from becoming a tangled, terrible mess: either use a slipknot to loop then over the lower bar of any hanger, or tuck each pair into its own sandwich bag and stash them in a box or drawer. In my actors' closets on set, I press one of those hanging shoe organizers that have clear pockets into service to store them. If you can afford the closet rail space, they are as close to perfect as tights and pantyhose storage is ever going to get until Cher's automated closet from *Clueless* becomes a reality.

ACKNOWLEDGMENTS

I'm the luckiest girl in the world to be able to work with everyone at Ten Speed Press again: my editor Kaitlin Ketchum (who always knows when an idea is right), Emma Rudolph (who got me over the biggest hurdles of this project), Dan Myers (who expertly managed production), Annie Marino and Emma Campion (who turned my words into the gem you are holding), and Daniel Wikey and Kristin Casemore (who make darn sure the whole world hears about this book)! Many thanks are also in order to Julia Kuo for the adorable illustrations.

I also owe a huge debt of gratitude to my family: my mom Jackie, my dad Doug, and my brother Paul, who always acted excited as I regaled them in excruciating detail about every single development of this book. And a very special thank you goes to my #1 human, Tommy Blacha. Anything funny you just read is a direct result of his sense of humor.

But the real MVPs here are my readers and Internet pals. Some of my best material was inspired by you, but I owe a special shout-out to Claire Denise for asking me how to rock a scarf "in that cute, jaunty way, both emotionally AND literally," as well as to Chelsei M. for wondering aloud how to wear accessories on the job "without feeling as if you suddenly decided to wear a novelty foam cowboy hat with your regular work outfit." I'm so grateful to every one of you, and I'd be nowhere without your support.

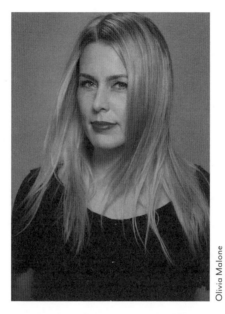

Olivia Malone

ABOUT THE AUTHOR

Alison Freer is a costume designer from Texas living and working in Hollywood. She got her start in fashion working at the mall, selling every type of accessory there is, from costume jewelry to shoes to designer handbags. She is a contributing writer on accessories, style, and how to shop the internet for *New York Magazine*, and the author of the *New York Times* best-seller *How To Get Dressed*. You can follow her on Instagram @AlisonFreer, on Twitter @AlisonVFreer, and on Facebook @AlisonFreerAuthor.

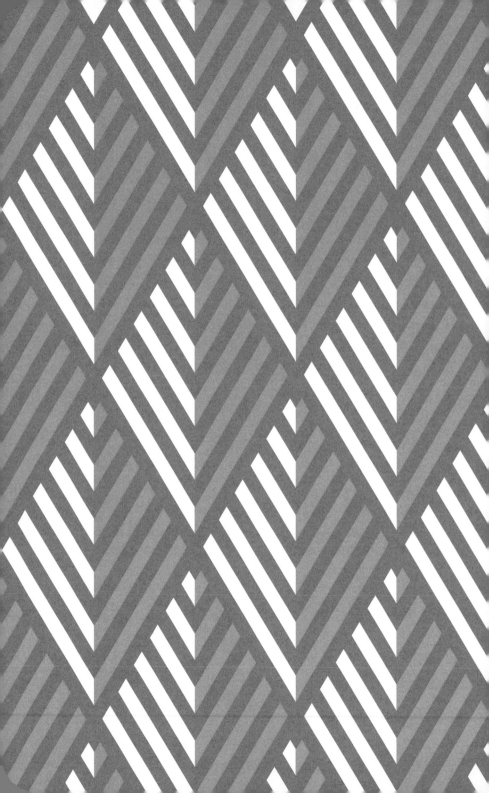

INDEX

Library of Congress Cataloging-in-Publication Data

Names: Freer, Alison, author.
Title: The accessory handbook : a costume designer's secrets for buying,
    wearing, and caring for accessories / by Alison Freer.
Description: First edition. | California : Ten Speed Press, [2018] | Includes
    index.
Identifiers: LCCN 2017056454 | ISBN 9780399580802 (trade pbk.)
Subjects: LCSH: Dress accessories.
Classification: LCC TT649.8 .F745 2018 | DDC 646/.3--dc23
LC record available at https://lccn.loc.gov/2017056454

Trade Paperback ISBN: 978-0-399-58080-2
eBook ISBN: 978-0-399-58081-9

Printed in China

Design by Annie Marino

10 9 8 7 6 5 4 3 2 1

First Edition